BRAIDS, BUNS, *and* TWISTS!

Step-by-Step Tutorials for 82 Fabulous Hairstyles

CHRISTINA BUTCHER

CHRONICLE BOOKS
SAN FRANCISCO

First published in the United States of America in 2013 by
Chronicle Books LLC.

Copyright © 2013 by RotoVision SA.
All rights reserved. No part of this book may be reproduced in any form
without written permission from the publisher.

Library of Congress Cataloging-in-Publication Data available.

ISBN: 978-1-4521-2484-1

Manufactured in China.

Cover designed by Kayla Ferriera.

Commissioning Editor: Isheeta Mustafi
Assistant Editor: Tamsin Richardson
Editor: Diane Leyman
Art Director: Emily Portnoi
Art Editor: Jennifer Osborne
Book layout: FentonForeman
Illustrations: Peters & Zabransky

Every effort has been made to contact owners of copyright material
produced in this book. In the event of a copyright query, please contact
the publisher.

10 9 8 7 6 5 4

Chronicle Books LLC
680 Second Street
San Francisco, CA 94107
www.chroniclebooks.com

This book is dedicated to Dad.
I miss you.

CONTENTS

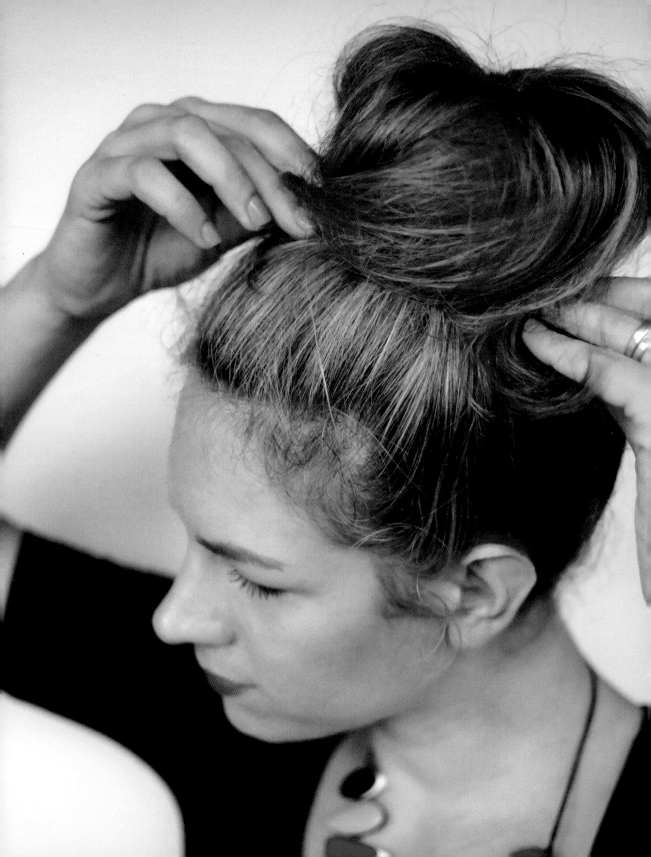

INTRODUCTION

Hello and welcome to *Braids, Buns, and Twists! Step-by-Step Tutorials for 82 Fabulous Hairstyles*. This book puts all the tools at your disposal so that you'll never have another bad hair day. Ever!

Have you found yourself in the same hair rut, day in, day out? Have you had enough of wearing your hair the same way since . . . forever? Are you trying to grow out your hair, but looking for fun ways to wear it in the meantime? There's nothing worse than being in hair limbo, and that's where this book can help. There are enough styles and variations within these pages to give you a different hairstyle every day of the week for almost a quarter of the year—the only downside is that you might get tired of people asking how you did your hair!

This book guides you through each style so that you can make the most of your best accessory: your hair. Chapters are organized by broad hairstyle: Ponytails; Braids; Buns, Knots, and Twists; and Bouffants. Each hairstyle entry tells you what's involved and where the style comes from and offers examples for when and where it might work best. Each style is given a difficulty rating, and you'll find tips and ideas on how to vary the style and what accessories to try. A list of styling tools and easy-to-follow, illustrated step-by-step tutorials make creating the styles simple, and beautiful photography shows how these styles look and work in real life. At the back of the book you'll also find a resources chapter, which details hairstyling tools, schools and further education, and a glossary.

For me, discovering I could do so much with my hair really helped my confidence. I struggled for years to understand how to deal with my own hair, and for a long time I hated it. Since developing the twist and pin technique (see pages 142–143), and learning how to treat my hair properly, I have finally come to love my hair. Now, when I see people trying out new styles in their own hair, I find it so inspiring.

Braids, Buns, and Twists! is here to help you practice and master all the techniques you need so that you can learn to love your hair too. This book shows how I create all my styles, and I know it won't be long before you love your hair just as much as I love mine. Your hair will become an exciting new part of your wardrobe that you can customize to go with whatever you're wearing and wherever you're going.

Enjoy the confidence your hair will bring. If I can do it, I know you can too!

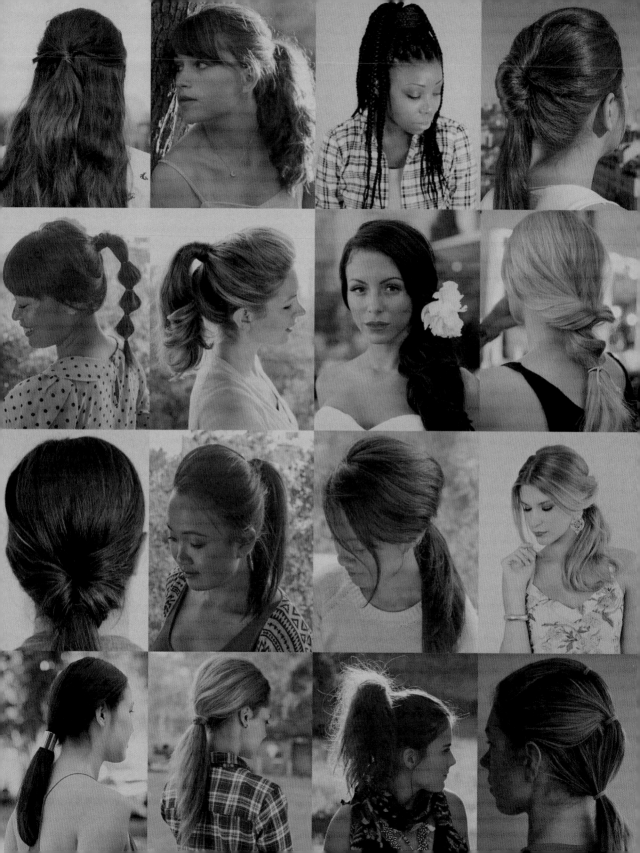

CHAPTER 1
PONYTAILS

QUIFFED PONYTAIL
THE LOOK

The quiffed ponytail is a fun hairstyle that transforms a plain pony into something special—it's a chic look but with just enough sass. To create this style, you'll tease the front and top of your hair to add height and volume. This hairstyle adds length to a shorter face and evokes a retro feel.

DIFFICULTY LEVEL
Easy

IDEAL HAIR LENGTH
Long

HAIR EXTENSIONS NEEDED?
No, but you can use a ponytail extension on shorter hair.

ASSISTANCE NEEDED?
No

ACCESSORIES
The quiff acts as a kind of accessory so you don't need to add any more. A scarf or bow on the ponytail can add a retro twist.

TRY THIS
Vary your look by experimenting with curly or straight hair. You can also twist the ponytail up into a ballerina bun (see pages 156–157) to make this great style into a cute updo.

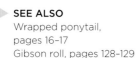

SEE ALSO
Wrapped ponytail, pages 16–17
Gibson roll, pages 128–129

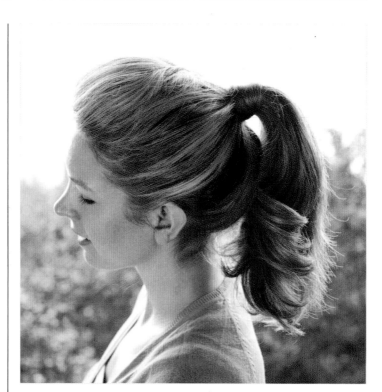

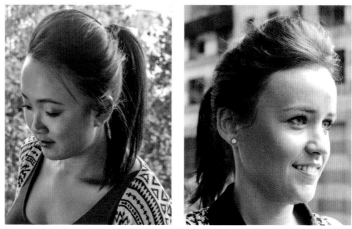

Top: Hairstyling and modeling by Christina Butcher, photography by Xiaohan Shen.
Bottom left: Hairstyling and photography by Christina Butcher, modeling by Adeline Er.
Bottom right: Hairstyling by Christina Butcher, photography by Xiaohan Shen, modeling by Sinead Brady.

HOW TO GET IT

WHAT YOU NEED

- Brush
- Teasing comb (optional)
- Bobby pins
- Hair elastic

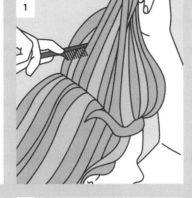

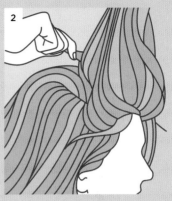

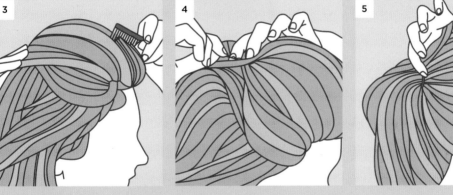

1-2. Lift the section of hair on the top of your head and begin backcombing your hair. Tease to create volume using a brush or teasing comb, starting at the crown and moving forward in sections toward your hairline.

3. Gently comb the top of your hair back over the teased quiff to smooth it and create the quiff shape.

4. Use a bobby pin just behind the quiff to secure it in place. Cross your bobby pins in an X shape for added hold.

5. Gather the rest of your hair up into a ponytail at the back of your head or place your ponytail a little higher, near your crown. Use an elastic to match your hair color, or wrap a small piece of hair around the elastic to hide it.

TOP TIP

If your hair is fine or soft, you'll need to use some product to hold the quiff and add volume. Before starting, apply mousse through your hair and blow-dry to add texture. You can also use hairspray to help hold the quiff in place, or use a sea salt product, which gives friction and helps to add volume.

HIGH CROWN PONYTAIL
THE LOOK

Ponytails that sit high on your crown have a fun, flirty feel. A sleek, high ponytail will swing as you walk, and this simple style looks effortlessly chic. Although it has a more relaxed feel, a high crown ponytail is still controlled enough to be work-appropriate, especially if you're going out in the evening or have an important meeting or interview during the day. The key to this look is to keep your hair smooth up to the ponytail. For a more youthful, sporty style, keep the finish a little loose and flyaway.

DIFFICULTY LEVEL
Easy

IDEAL HAIR LENGTH
Long

HAIR EXTENSIONS NEEDED?
No, but you can use a ponytail extension on shorter hair.

ASSISTANCE NEEDED?
No

ACCESSORIES
If you need to pin back your bangs, a jeweled pin is the only accessory required. Metallic hair cuffs can also take this sleek ponytail one step further.

TRY THIS
Wear this ponytail super sleek with straight hair, or give it a cute, sporty look with a little curl at the ends. This will encourage the pony to bounce as you walk.

▶ **SEE ALSO**
Stacked ponytail, pages 26–27
Donut bun, pages 118–119

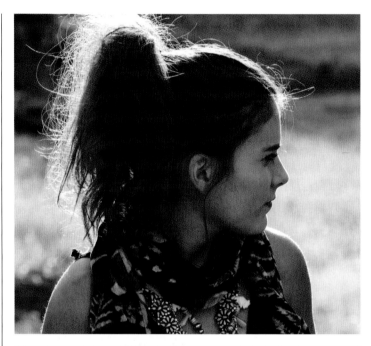

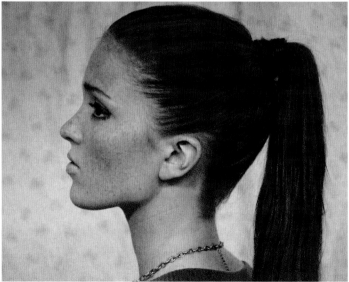

Top: Hairstyling, photography, and modeling by Emily Goswick.
Bottom: Hairstyling, photography, and modeling by Emily M. Meyers/The Freckled Fox.

HOW TO GET IT

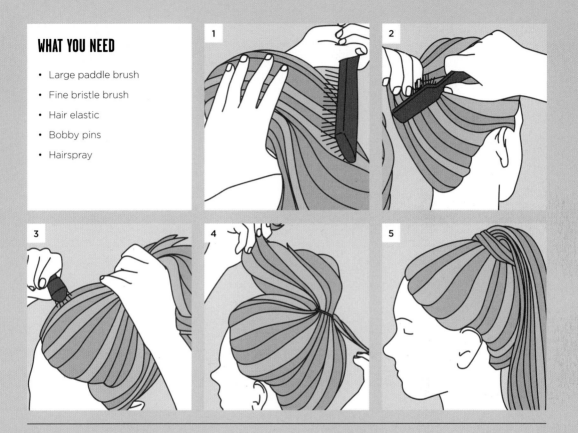

WHAT YOU NEED

- Large paddle brush
- Fine bristle brush
- Hair elastic
- Bobby pins
- Hairspray

1. Brush your hair to remove any knots and smooth it out. Use a large paddle brush to gather all your hair at the crown.

2-3. Next, take a smaller bristle brush to smooth all your hair back into a ponytail. You can use the bigger paddle brush, but you'll have more control with a smaller brush.

4. Secure your ponytail with an elastic. Ensure it is a tight fit so that your ponytail stays up high on or near the crown of your head. Take a small section of hair from your ponytail and wrap it around the base of your ponytail to hide the hair elastic. Use a bobby pin to secure it underneath your ponytail so that it won't be seen.

5. Use hairspray to tame any flyaways and keep your ponytail looking sleek, or allow some of the flyaways to stay to give the style a more casual, relaxed look.

TOP TIP

To keep this ponytail super sleek, use this backstage styling secret: spray hairspray on a toothbrush and use it to brush back any baby-fine hairs and flyaways. This technique won't overload your hair with hairspray, but will keep all those fine hairs in place.

13

CURLY PONYTAIL
THE LOOK

This hairstyle is perfect for those with naturally curly hair, but you can also use a curling iron to create your own curls. The secret to this style is using a hair bungee instead of an elastic to secure the ponytail in place. A hair bungee is a piece of elastic with a hook at each end which wraps around your ponytail so that you don't need to pull your curls through a tight band. This leaves your curls in much better shape and less frizzy than with a normal hair elastic.

DIFFICULTY LEVEL
Easy

IDEAL HAIR LENGTH
Medium to long

HAIR EXTENSIONS NEEDED?
No

ASSISTANCE NEEDED?
No

ACCESSORIES
Pretty up your ponytail with a flower corsage, or keep it simple with a headband to keep your bangs away from your face.

TRY THIS
This ponytail can be worn in any position: it all depends on your curls and how you like to wear them. Try putting your hair up into a high crown ponytail (see pages 12–13), gathering your curls at your neck for a low ponytail, or sweeping them over your shoulder for a side pony.

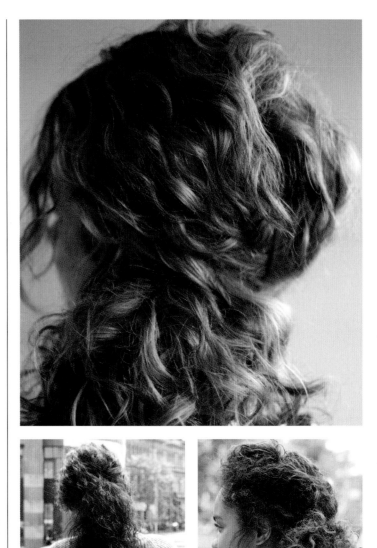

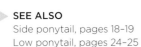

▶ **SEE ALSO**
Side ponytail, pages 18–19
Low ponytail, pages 24–25

Top: Hairstyling, photography, and modeling by Christina Butcher.
Bottom left: Hairstyling by Christina Butcher, photography by Xiaohan Shen, modeling by Delphine Peyriere.
Bottom right: Hairstyling by Christina Butcher, photography by Xiaohan Shen, modeling by Ornella Joaquim.

HOW TO GET IT

WHAT YOU NEED

- Curl cream or gel (optional)
- Blow-dryer and diffuser attachment (optional)
- 1-inch curling iron (optional)
- Hair bungee
- Bobby pin (optional)

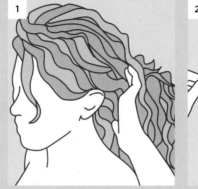

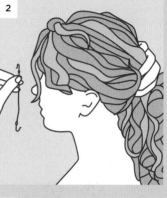

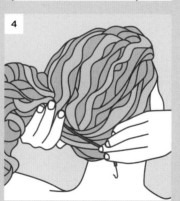

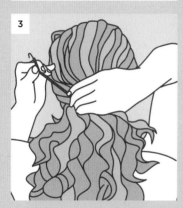

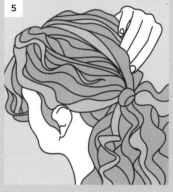

1. Style your curls as you would normally wear them. For naturally curly hair, use a curl cream or gel to and let your curls dry naturally. You can use a diffuser attachment on your blow-dryer to dry them more quickly. For straight hair, use a 1-inch curling iron to curl your hair. Work in small sections, starting from underneath and working up to the top of your hair. Let the curls cool and gently shake them with your fingertips to create a more natural look.

2. Use your fingers to gather your hair into a ponytail. It's best to avoid brushes and combs, as they break up curls and cause them to frizz.

3–4. Take your hair bungee and hook it into the base of your ponytail. Wind it around your hair until it is tight enough to hold. Place the other hook in your hair to secure your ponytail.

5. Gently pull at the hair around the bungee to soften the look. Your curls should hide the bungee, or you can pin a small piece of hair around to cover it.

TOP TIP

To keep your curls looking defined and frizz-free, don't use a brush or comb on dry hair. Instead, use your fingers to shape your ponytail. After washing, don't rub your curls with a towel, as this will cause them to frizz. Instead, just squeeze the excess water out with a towel and dry with a blow-dryer.

WRAPPED PONYTAIL
THE LOOK

This wrapped ponytail is the perfect style if you have long hair and find it difficult to keep your ponytail in place. It's a casual yet sophisticated hairstyle that works from day to night. By leaving out the top section of hair, you'll find it easier to put the remainder of your hair up. The top section is then wrapped around the base of the ponytail in a twisting motion. You angle your hair down as you wrap, and then your ponytail is pinned flat against the back of your head.

DIFFICULTY LEVEL
Medium

IDEAL HAIR LENGTH
Medium to long

HAIR EXTENSIONS NEEDED?
No, but you can use a ponytail extension on shorter hair.

ASSISTANCE NEEDED?
No

ACCESSORIES
Your hair acts as an accessory in this hairstyle, wrapping around your ponytail to create a twist. A jeweled clip or flower can be pinned into the side of the twist to add a more detailed look for nighttime.

TRY THIS
Adjust the position of the ponytail to give this hairstyle a different look. For instance, you could tie a really high ponytail or place it lower on the back of your head.

> **SEE ALSO**
> Top knot bun, pages 116–117
> French twist, pages 130–131

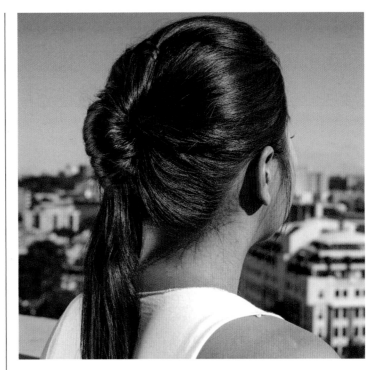

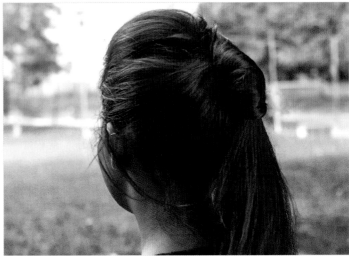

Top: Hairstyling and photography by Christina Butcher, modeling by An Ly.
Bottom: Hairstyling and photography by Christina Butcher, modeling by Nicole Jeyaraj.

HOW TO GET IT

WHAT YOU NEED

- Brush
- Hair clip
- Hair elastic
- Bobby pins
- Hairspray (optional)

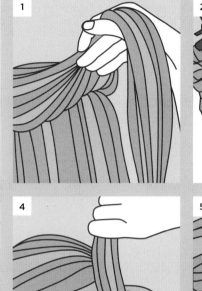

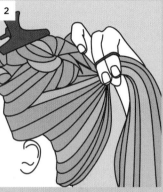

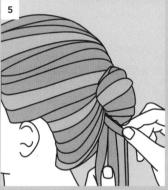

1. Brush your hair to remove any knots before you begin. Take a section of hair at the top of your head to your crown and clip it up and out of the way.

2. Gather the remainder of your hair into a ponytail at your crown. Try to place the base of the ponytail close to the edge of the section you clipped up at the top. Secure your ponytail with a hair elastic.

3. Next, unclip the top section of hair and adjust the front to sit in a small pompadour shape. Use a bobby pin to secure in place just above your ponytail.

4. Wrap the remainder of the top section of hair around your ponytail. Stay as close to the base of your ponytail as possible to avoid the hair sliding down as you wrap it around. Secure the end of the wrapped section with a bobby pin.

5. Flatten your ponytail against the back of your head and use bobby pins to secure it in place.

TOP TIP

To get a neat, smooth finish, hold the end of your ponytail while you adjust the wrapped section so that it sits flat against the back of your head. Angle your bobby pins diagonally, and for a stronger hold you can cross your pins in an X shape. Finish with hairspray to keep your ponytail in place.

SIDE PONYTAIL
THE LOOK

A casual twist on the traditional ponytail, wearing your hair to the side is an easy, everyday hairstyle. Many movie stars have been spotted sporting a side pony, making it a popular style all over again. The fun, asymmetrical angle is on-trend, yet this style still allows for a sleek finish. This ponytail works for both curly and straight hair and can be dressed up for an evening look. Covering your hair elastic with a section of hair gives it a seamless finish.

DIFFICULTY LEVEL
Easy

IDEAL HAIR LENGTH
Medium to long

HAIR EXTENSIONS NEEDED?
No

ASSISTANCE NEEDED?
No

ACCESSORIES
Wear flowers in your hair for a bohemian feel. Flower crowns or ponytail corsages are sweet accessories to turn this into a summer festival hairstyle or a style that begs for a day at the beach.

TRY THIS
If you have bangs, you can twist or braid them back to join the ponytail at the side of your head. Why not try a fishtail braid in your ponytail? Follow the tutorial on pages 50–51 to combine these two hairstyles.

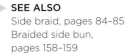
SEE ALSO
Side braid, pages 84–85
Braided side bun, pages 158–159

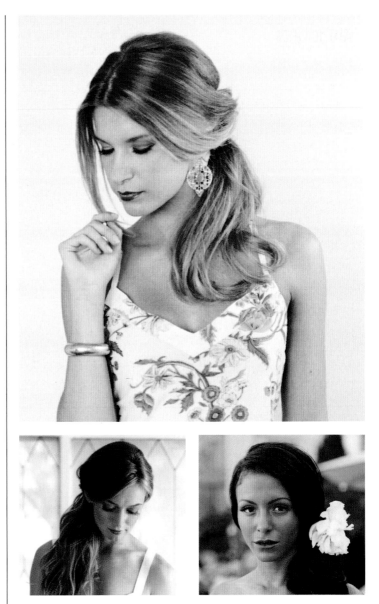

Top: Photograph courtesy of Plum Pretty Sugar. Hairstyling by Makeup 1011 and Katie M, photography by Marisa Holmes.
Bottom left: Hairstyling by Amber Rose Hair + Makeup, photography by Eliesa Johnson, wardrobe by Anne Kristine Lingerie, modeling by Lindsey.
Bottom right: Hairstyling by Flavia Carolina with Versa Artistry, photography by Heather Nan.

HOW TO GET IT

WHAT YOU NEED

- Brush
- Hair elastic
- Bobby pin

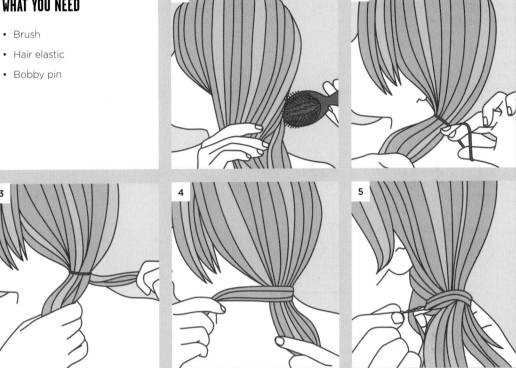

1. Brush your hair to remove any knots. Part your hair to the side.
2. Sweep all your hair over to the opposite side to your part and brush into a side ponytail. Secure your ponytail with a hair elastic.
3. Take a small section of hair from your ponytail.
4. Wrap the section of hair around your hair elastic.
5. Pin the end of the section underneath your ponytail with a bobby pin to keep it in place.

TOP TIP

Don't try to place your ponytail too high, as this will take away from the modern look you are trying to achieve. Instead, let your ponytail rest on your shoulder for a more casual look.

HALF PONYTAIL
THE LOOK

Create an elegant half-up, half-down hairstyle with the half ponytail, a classic style that suits so many situations. Because it's quick and easy to do, the half ponytail is perfect for relaxed social occasions, but has enough sophistication for a formal work or evening function. The half ponytail works with all hair types, from fine and straight to thick and curly. This style can be transformed from bohemian to modern with the right hair accessory.

DIFFICULTY LEVEL
Easy

IDEAL HAIR LENGTH
Medium to long

HAIR EXTENSIONS NEEDED?
No

ASSISTANCE NEEDED?
No

ACCESSORIES
Embellish this simple hairstyle with flowers, jeweled hairpins, or clips. Pin a bow at the back for a cute look, or use flowers to give it a bohemian feel.

TRY THIS
Combine the half ponytail with the flipped-over ponytail (see pages 22–23) to create a half-flip hairstyle.

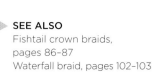

SEE ALSO
Fishtail crown braids, pages 86–87
Waterfall braid, pages 102–103

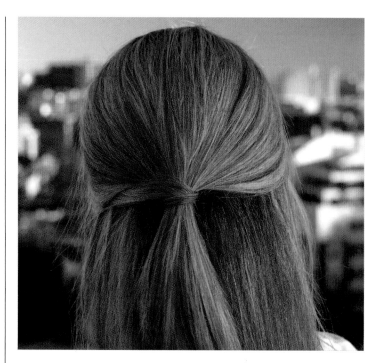

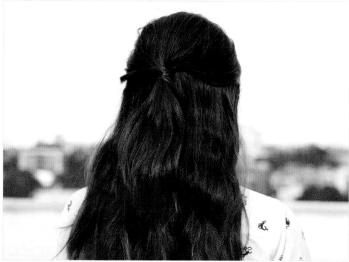

Top: Hairstyling, photography, and modeling by Christina Butcher.
Bottom: Hairstyling by Christina Butcher, photography by Xiaohan Shen, modeling by Sophia Phan.

HOW TO GET IT

WHAT YOU NEED

- Brush
- Clear hair elastic
- Bobby pins

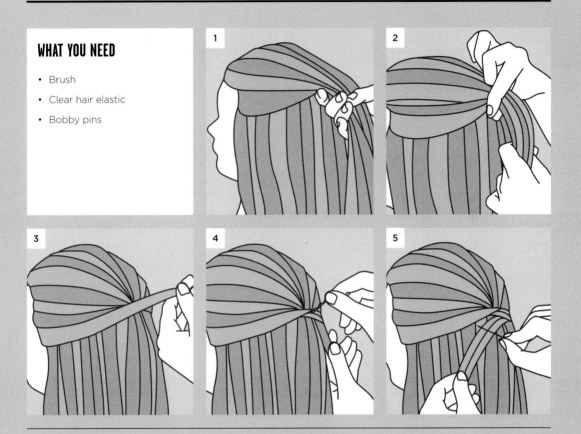

1. Part a straight line from just above your ears around the back of your head, and lift this top section up.

2. Secure this section with a hair elastic at the back of your head.

3. Take a small piece of hair from above your left ear and take it around the back to wrap around your hair elastic.

4. Pin the section of hair in place with a bobby pin.

5. Repeat on the right-hand side, bringing a small piece of hair over to hide your hair elastic, and pin in place.

TOP TIP

When pinning the pieces of hair over your hair elastic, hold your bobby pin vertically and push it up and slightly diagonally to keep it in place. Using small sections of hair to cover the hair elastic turns this style, often seen as utilitarian, into a more elegant and versatile look.

FLIPPED-OVER PONYTAIL
THE LOOK

Turn the classic ponytail style on its head with the flipped-over ponytail. By turning the base of the ponytail inside out and pushing it through itself, you can add body to your ponytail and give it a different dimension. The knot or bun that you're left with at the base of the ponytail is its own accessory, though a flower corsage or ribbon can be added for a touch of color. Perfect for school, work, or going out with friends, this style is a pretty alternative to a regular ponytail.

DIFFICULTY LEVEL
Easy

IDEAL HAIR LENGTH
Medium to long

HAIR EXTENSIONS NEEDED?
No

ASSISTANCE NEEDED?
No

ACCESSORIES
Use hair elastics that match the color of your hair to keep them inconspicuous. Add a pin or flower corsage in between the flip for an elegant or formal look.

TRY THIS
Combine the flipped-over ponytail with the half ponytail (see pages 20–21) for a pretty half-up style. You can also continue flipping your ponytail for a double- or triple-flip hairstyle. Combine this technique with the bobble ponytail (see pages 34–35) for an almost-braided ponytail look.

▶ **SEE ALSO**
Half ponytail, pages 20–21
Bobble ponytail, pages 34–35

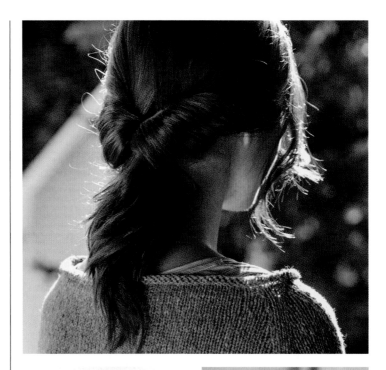

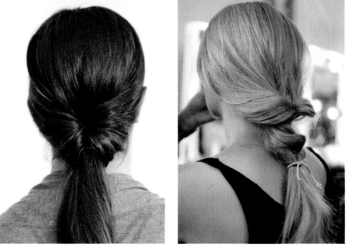

Top: Photograph courtesy of Brooklyn Tweed. Hairstyling by Véronik Avery, photography by Jared Flood, modeling by Stephanie Gelot.
Bottom left: Hairstyling and photography by Marie-Pierre Sander.
Bottom right: Hairstyling and photography by Christina Butcher, modeling by Fiana Stewart.

HOW TO GET IT

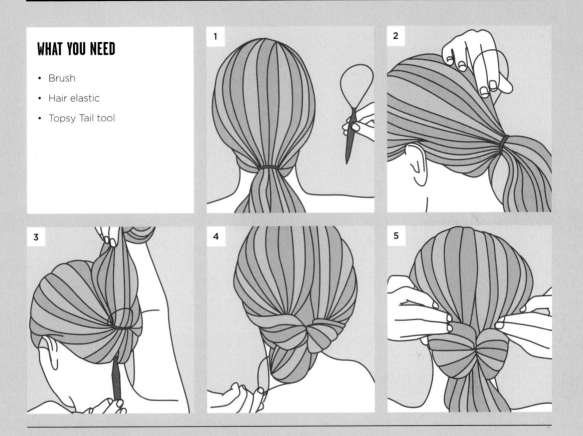

WHAT YOU NEED

- Brush
- Hair elastic
- Topsy Tail tool

1. Brush your hair to remove any knots. Gather your hair into a ponytail at the back of your head or sitting low above your neck and secure it with an elastic.

2. Take your Topsy Tail tool and place it in your hair above your ponytail elastic.

3. Pull your ponytail up through the loop of the Topsy Tail tool.

4. While holding the end of your ponytail up, pull the Topsy Tail down. You may need to adjust it as your hair elastic is flipped over. Keep pulling your hair down until it is all the way through.

5. Adjust the twisted sections to sit neatly.

TOP TIP

It's possible to do this style without the Topsy Tail: simply use your fingers to make a space above your hair elastic and flip your ponytail through. Alternatively, you can DIY your own tool with fabric-covered wire.

LOW PONYTAIL
THE LOOK

The low ponytail is an easy, elegant hairstyle that suits all sorts of occasions. This ponytail hangs low at the nape of your neck and leaves the back of your head looking sleek. It will also make your hair look longer than in a high ponytail, as your hair lays down the length of your back. More serious than the high crown ponytail, this classic hairstyle suits all hair types and lengths. You can keep it chic with a neat center part, or wear it with a deep side part for a more glamorous feel.

DIFFICULTY LEVEL
Easy

IDEAL HAIR LENGTH
Medium to long

HAIR EXTENSIONS NEEDED?
No, but you can use a ponytail extension on shorter hair.

ASSISTANCE NEEDED?
No

ACCESSORIES
With such a simple style, you can add any accessory to transform your look for any occasion.

TRY THIS
Changing your part will change the look of this hairstyle. You can wear a neat center part for a simple symmetrical look, a classic side part for a smart feel, or a sleek, deep side part for a glamorous nighttime look.

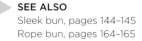 **SEE ALSO**
Sleek bun, pages 144–145
Rope bun, pages 164–165

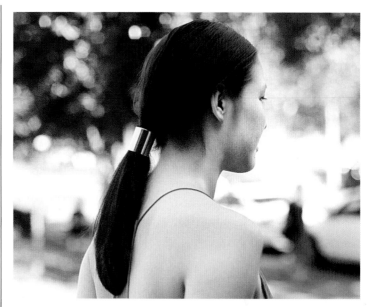

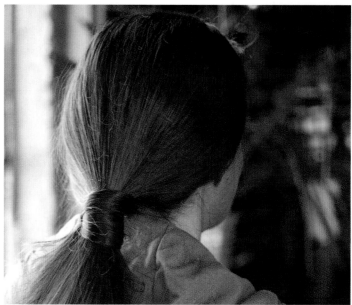

Top: Hairstyling by Christina Butcher, photography by Xiaohan Shen, modeling by Tash Williams.
Bottom: Hairstyling and photography by Christina Butcher, modeling by Emily Yeo.

HOW TO GET IT

WHAT YOU NEED

- Brush
- Tail comb (optional)
- Hair elastic
- Bobby pin
- Hairspray (optional)

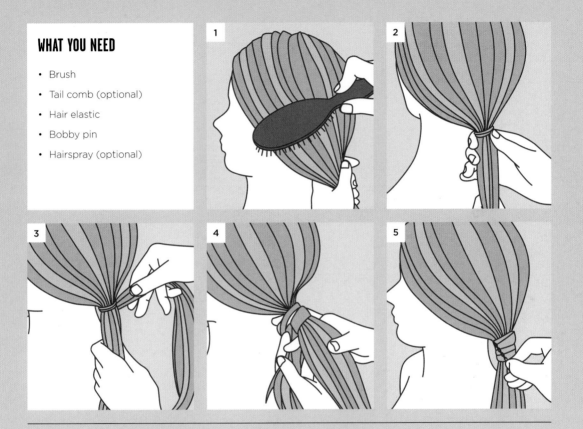

1. Brush your hair to remove any knots. Decide where you want to part your hair. Follow your natural part, or use a tail comb to make a new part line. Brush all your hair back into a low ponytail, sitting right on the nape of your neck.

2. Secure with a hair elastic and adjust your hair so that it sits tight to your head.

3-5. Cover your hair elastic by taking a small piece of hair from your ponytail and wrapping it around the base of your ponytail. Pin the end in place with a bobby pin.

TOP TIP

To keep your ponytail looking sleek as it lays down your back, spray hairspray onto the teeth of a comb and run it through the loose hair. This is a great stylist's trick; it doesn't overload and stiffen the ponytail with too much product but still gives the hair hold and stops flyaways.

STACKED PONYTAIL
THE LOOK

This sleek, sectioned ponytail is an elegant take on the classic low ponytail. Recently seen on Fashion Week catwalks, this style can take your everyday ponytail from ordinary to extraordinary. Good for both daytime and nighttime wear, this pony style maintains your hair length while at the same time giving it a stylishly simple look.

DIFFICULTY LEVEL
Easy

IDEAL HAIR LENGTH
Long

HAIR EXTENSIONS NEEDED?
No, but you can use a ponytail extension on medium-length hair.

ASSISTANCE NEEDED?
No

ACCESSORIES
Use clear elastics for an elegant ponytail, or try colored hair ties for a fun variation. For nighttime you could add a jeweled ponytail clip at the base.

TRY THIS
You can create a stack of four or five ponytails by taking smaller sections down the back of your head. You could even continue down your ponytail the same as in the bobble ponytail (see pages 34–35).

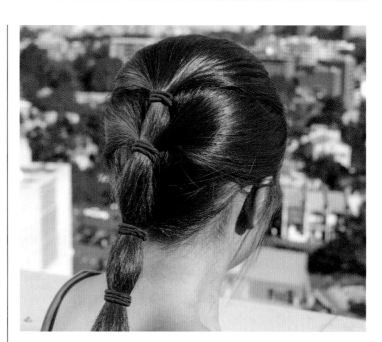

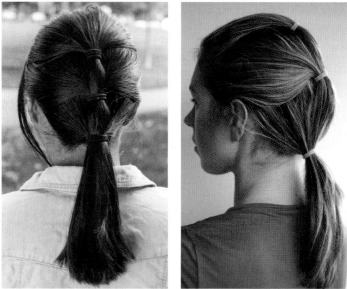

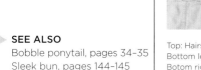

▶ **SEE ALSO**
Bobble ponytail, pages 34–35
Sleek bun, pages 144–145

Top: Hairstyling and photography by Christina Butcher, modeling by Adeline Er.
Bottom left: Hairstyling and photography by Christina Butcher, modeling by Willa Zheng.
Botom right: Hairstyling, photography, and modeling by Christina Butcher.

HOW TO GET IT

WHAT YOU NEED

- Brush
- 3 hair elastics
- Hair serum
- Hairspray

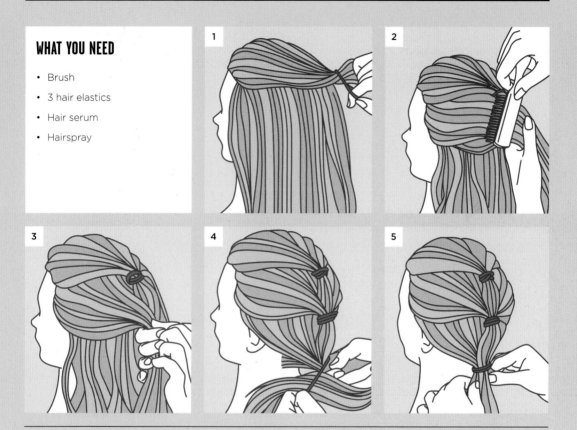

1. Make a ponytail at the top of your head with a one-third section of hair, and secure with an elastic.

2. Brush back the next section of hair at ear level to create a ponytail at the back of your head, incorporating the first ponytail.

3. Secure this second section with a hair elastic.

4. Gather all your hair into a ponytail at the nape of your neck and secure with an elastic.

5. Smooth your ponytail with serum and finish with a light mist of hairspray to catch any flyaways.

TOP TIP

Spray hairspray onto your brush, rather than your hair, then lightly brush to catch those fine flyaway hairs. If you have layers, curl the ends of your hair under so that they don't stick out of your ponytail.

TWIST-OVER PONYTAIL
THE LOOK

Put beautiful detail into your hair with the twist-over ponytail. Creating small rope twists that join into the main ponytail adds a cosmopolitan, chic look to the regular ponytail style. Perfect for the social scene—just get ready for everyone asking how you did it! This twist-over ponytail works if you have layers in your hair, as long as they reach your ponytail. If you don't have a lot of hair, a ponytail extension will give you a fuller look.

DIFFICULTY LEVEL
Medium

IDEAL HAIR LENGTH
Medium to long

HAIR EXTENSIONS NEEDED?
No, but you can use a ponytail extension on shorter hair.

ASSISTANCE NEEDED?
No

ACCESSORIES
You don't really need to add accessories to this look, as there is enough pretty detail in the twisted sections. This low hairstyle is perfect under a hat or headband.

TRY THIS
Instead of twisting each section, try simple braids. They will add more texture to the style. Alternatively, split the side sections into more subsections—try four or even five small twisted sections to add into the ponytail to create a more intricate look.

▶ **SEE ALSO**
   Flipped-over ponytail, pages 22–23
   Figure-8 braid, pages 76–77

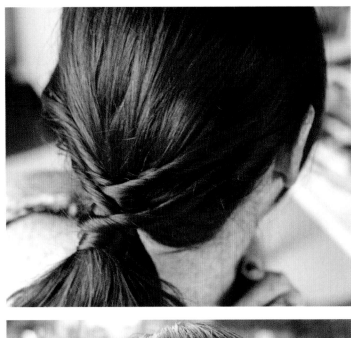

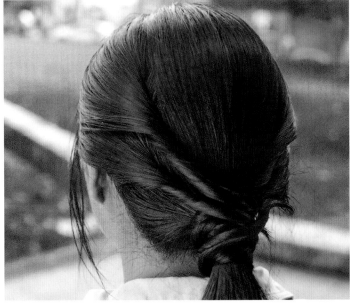

Top: Hairstyling and photography by Christina Butcher, modeling by Monica Richmond.
Bottom: Hairstyling and photography by Christina Butcher, modeling by Willa Zheng.

HOW TO GET IT

WHAT YOU NEED

- Brush
- Hair clips
- Hair elastic
- Bobby pins

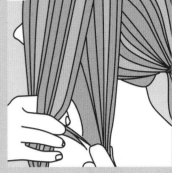

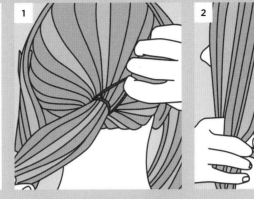

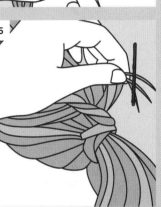

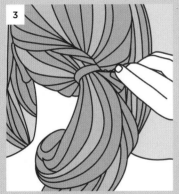

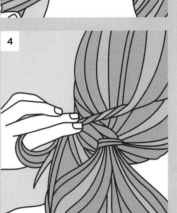

1. Brush your hair through to remove any knots or tangles. Clip away two medium-sized sections of hair, one on either side of your face. Put the rest of your hair in a ponytail and secure with a hair elastic.

2. Separate each side section into three equal parts.

3. Starting with the lowest section, twist the hair into a rope and then wrap it around your ponytail. Secure the end with a bobby pin.

4. Repeat on the other side, then go on to the middle section, and so on.

5. Continue twisting each section and pin in place around your ponytail with bobby pins until you're done.

TOP TIP

A trick for keeping your hair in place is to tease the end of each section, wrap it around the elastic, and then pin in place. Putting the pin on the end of your hair first will make this much easier to do. You could also curl your hair slightly before wrapping it around the ponytail, as this helps keep the ends from sticking out.

1960s PONYTAIL
THE LOOK

Channel your inner Bardot with this retro-inspired ponytail. The crown is lightly teased to create volume and the ponytail sits low at the back of the head. The curved ends to the ponytail give this style that '60s glam look.

DIFFICULTY LEVEL
Easy

IDEAL HAIR LENGTH
Long

HAIR EXTENSIONS NEEDED?
No, but you can use a ponytail extension on medium-length hair.

ASSISTANCE NEEDED?
No

ACCESSORIES
If you have bangs you can use a pretty pin to clip them back. Sideswept bangs will embrace that '60s feel.

TRY THIS
Keep it loose and messy for a Brigitte Bardot feel, and wear with winged eyeliner. For a chic, evening updo, twist the ponytail into a chignon at the nape of your neck.

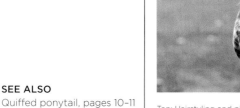

SEE ALSO
Quiffed ponytail, pages 10–11
Classic 1960s bouffant, pages 176–177

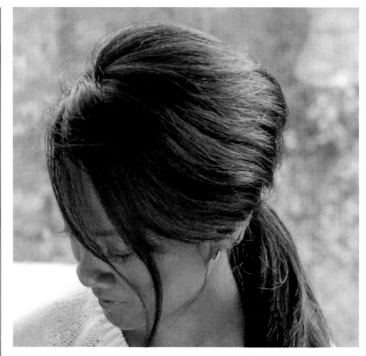

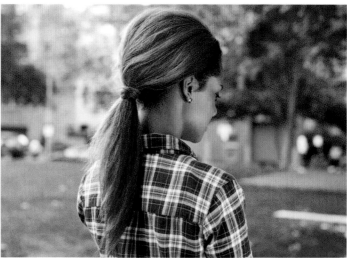

Top: Hairstyling and photography by Christina Butcher, modeling by Patricia Almario.
Bottom: Hairstyling by Christina Butcher, photography by Xiaohan Shen, modeling by Dorothy Jean Joly.

HOW TO GET IT

WHAT YOU NEED

- Bristle brush or comb
- Hairspray (optional)
- Hair elastic
- Bobby pins

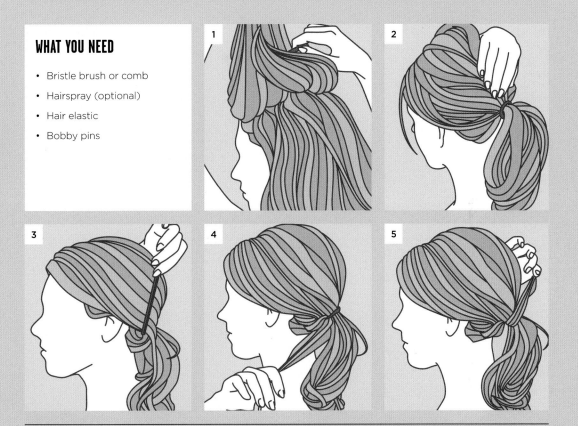

1. Separate your hair into top and bottom sections. Create volume and a bouffant shape with the top section by teasing at the crown of your head using a comb or bristle brush. Add a little hairspray if you need extra hold.

2. Gather all your hair into a low ponytail and secure with a hair elastic. Don't pull the hair too tightly, as you want to keep as much volume as possible in the crown area. Gently pull at the top of your ponytail to loosen the hair and create a 1960s silhouette.

3. Using the bristle brush or comb, smooth over the top section of hair to create a rounder shape.

4. Take a small piece of hair from the base of your ponytail and wrap it around your hair elastic to cover it.

5. Secure the ends of the wrapped hair underneath with a bobby pin.

TOP TIP

It's important to start this style with a strong base and, depending on your hair type, you will need some product to create volume. Try a volumizer or mousse in towel-dried hair and blow-dry with a round brush. If your hair is naturally wavy or curly, second-day hair will also hold this style well.

MESSY PONYTAIL
THE LOOK

There's an art to the effortlessly stylish, messy ponytail. It's the height of Parisian chic and is a standout for that done-on-purpose, on-trend messy look. To get the right kind of messy ponytail, you need to start with roughly textured hair, which is achievable in hair a day after washing or by using product. This style works well in fine, straight hair but looks great in curly or thick hair too.

DIFFICULTY LEVEL
Easy

IDEAL HAIR LENGTH
Medium to long

HAIR EXTENSIONS NEEDED?
No

ASSISTANCE NEEDED?
No

ACCESSORIES
Keep this looking effortless by staying low-key with your accessories. A thin ribbon or small neutral flower corsage is all this style needs.

TRY THIS
Move your ponytail around—try a high messy ponytail or fix it low at the nape of your neck. Using the softness you get from this style, transform your messy ponytail into a side pony for an asymmetrical look.

 SEE ALSO
Messy low bun, pages 126–127
Messy side bun, pages 138–139

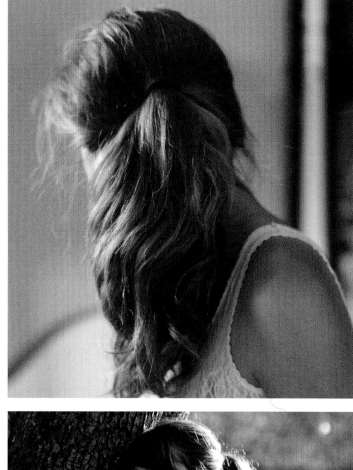

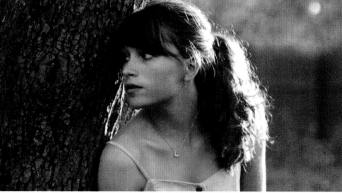

Top: Hairstyling, photography, and modeling by Alison Titus.
Bottom: Hairstyling, photography, and modeling by Alison Titus.

HOW TO GET IT

WHAT YOU NEED

- Comb (optional)
- Hair elastic
- Bobby pins (optional)
- Sea salt spray or matte
  styling powders (optional)

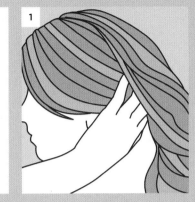

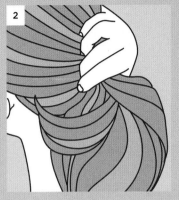

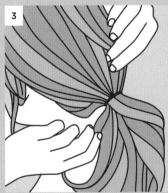

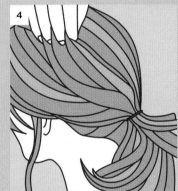

1. Put down your brush—you want to keep this look as messy as possible! You can use a comb to lightly backcomb at your roots to add some volume, but this is optional.

2. Use your fingers to loosely gather your hair up into a mid-height ponytail at the back of your head.

3. Secure your hair with a hair elastic.

4. Gently pull the hair above the elastic so that it isn't tight against your head. Rub your hair between your fingers a little to encourage more texture.

TOP TIP

This messy style works best in second-day hair, when your hair has more texture. If you want to recreate the look of second-day hair, use a sea salt spray or matte styling powders to add some grit and texture. This will replicate the perfect messy texture you're looking for.

BOBBLE PONYTAIL
THE LOOK

With such a distinctive shape, the sectioned bobble ponytail is fun but sleek and is so easy to do. Puff out each section of the ponytail to give it a unique look. This style combines the functionality of keeping your hair well and truly under control with a cute look that's perfect for a day out with friends.

DIFFICULTY LEVEL
Easy

IDEAL HAIR LENGTH
Long

HAIR EXTENSIONS NEEDED?
No, but you can use a ponytail extension on shorter hair.

ASSISTANCE NEEDED?
No

ACCESSORIES
For a more streamlined look, use hair elastics that match your hair color. Alternatively, why not try metallic hair elastics or hair cuffs as a feature, or use colored hair ties for a fun finish.

TRY THIS
This hairstyle is really effective in straight hair, though it can also be worn in wavy or curly hair. Why not combine the bobble ponytail with the stacked ponytail (see pages 26–27)? Section your hair down the back of your head and continue into a low bobble ponytail at the nape of your neck. You can also wear this hairstyle to the side or twist it into a top knot bun for added texture.

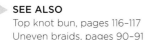

SEE ALSO
Top knot bun, pages 116–117
Uneven braids, pages 90–91

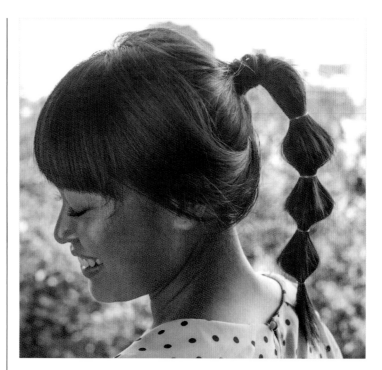

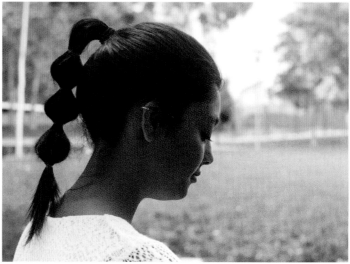

Top: Hairstyling and photography by Christina Butcher, modeling by Carolyn Mach.
Bottom: Hairstyling and photography by Christina Butcher, modeling by Nicole Jeyaraj.

HOW TO GET IT

WHAT YOU NEED

- Brush
- 4–6 hair elastics (depending on the length of your hair)

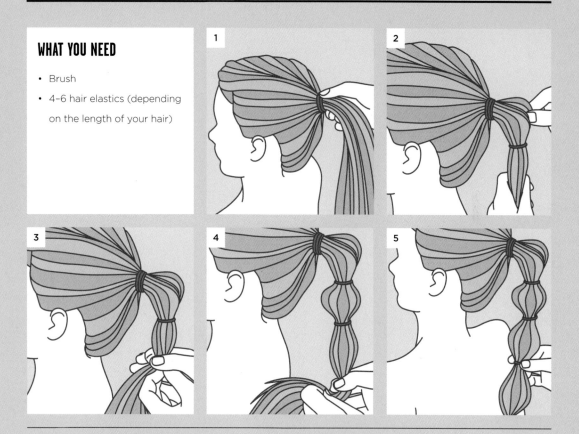

1. Brush your hair to remove any knots. Gather all your hair into a ponytail at the back of your head and secure with an elastic. You can place the ponytail higher on the crown of your head if you're after a bouncier look.

2. Next, take a hair elastic and place it around your ponytail about 2 inches from the base of your ponytail.

3. Continue placing hair elastics in equal measures down the length of your ponytail.

4. Keep going!

5. When you're done, gently pull at each section of hair to stretch it out and emphasize the shape.

TOP TIP

Gently pulling at each section of hair not only emphasizes the distinctive shape of this ponytail, but also makes your hair look thicker.

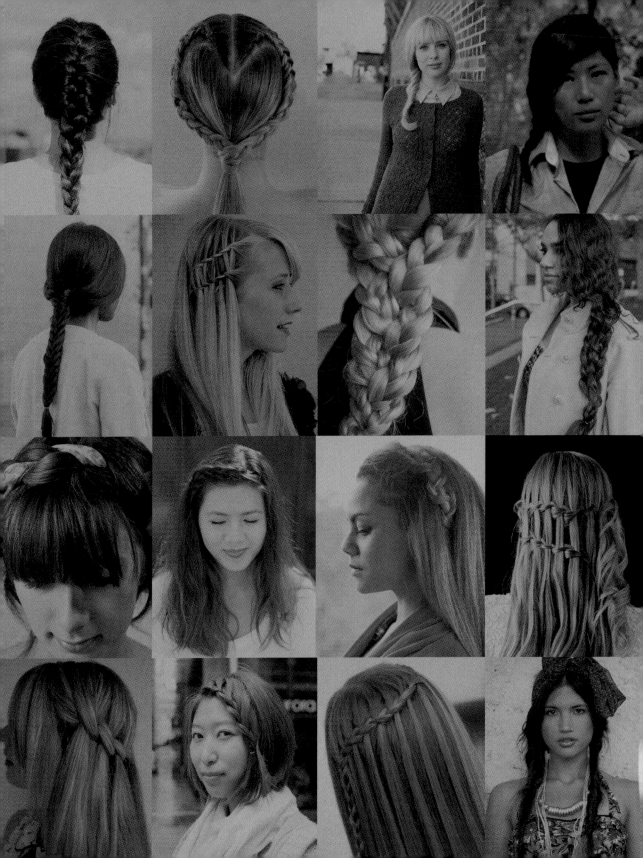

CHAPTER 2
BRAIDS

BASIC BRAID
THE LOOK

The basic braid is also known as a plait. It is the main building block you'll use for all braiding styles, but it's also a beautiful hairstyle on its own. It involves weaving three sections of hair together and repeating this process to form the braid. This really is one of the most versatile techniques and looks great in all hair types. It can be used in so many different ways, as you'll see throughout this chapter.

DIFFICULTY LEVEL
Easy

IDEAL HAIR LENGTH
Medium to long

HAIR EXTENSIONS NEEDED?
No

ASSISTANCE NEEDED?
No

ACCESSORIES
Team the braid with a ribbon or bow for a cute finish, or use flowers for a bohemian look.

TRY THIS
You can wear the basic braid anywhere in your hair. Wear it to the back or over your shoulder to the side. Combine this with the half ponytail (see pages 20–21) for a half-up braid, or with the high crown ponytail (see pages 12–13) for a high braided ponytail.

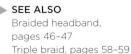

SEE ALSO
Braided headband, pages 46–47
Triple braid, pages 58–59

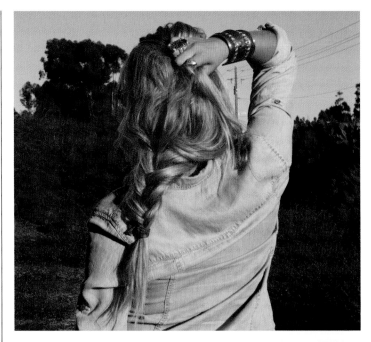

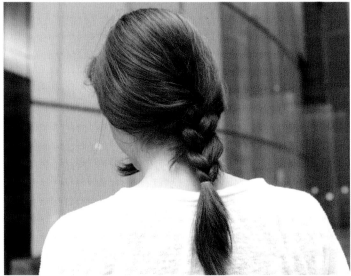

Top: Hairstyling, photography, and modeling by Emily Goswick.
Bottom: Hairstyling by Christina Butcher, photography by Xiaohan Shen, modeling by Laura Muheim.

HOW TO GET IT

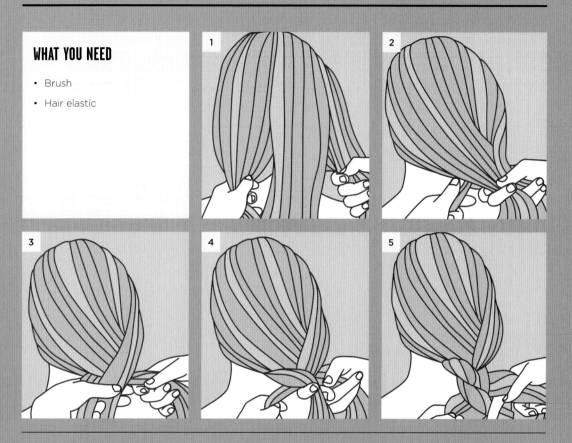

WHAT YOU NEED

- Brush
- Hair elastic

1. Brush your hair to remove any knots and split your hair into three equal pieces.

2. Take the piece on the left and cross it over the middle. Next, take the piece on the right and cross it over the left (now middle) piece. You'll start to see the braid forming.

3. Take the section now on the left and cross it over the middle and then repeat again, bringing the right over the left (now middle).

4. As you continue down, bring each outer piece over the middle to keep forming the braid.

5. When you're finished, secure the end of your hair with an elastic.

TOP TIP

Using small clear elastics will help when creating braided hairstyles, as the band won't show through the finished upstyle. Pull gently at the sides of your braid to loosen it and stretch it out. This will make your hair look thicker and emphasize the shape.

REVERSE BRAID
THE LOOK

The reverse braid is exactly that—the reverse of a basic braid. It's sometimes called the backward braid or inside-out braid. The technique is the same as the basic braid, but rather than bringing the sections over to form a braid, they move underneath to create a reverse braid. This technique shows off the structure of the braid more than a basic braid and stands away from the head. It works well in all hair types.

DIFFICULTY LEVEL
Easy

IDEAL HAIR LENGTH
Medium to long

HAIR EXTENSIONS NEEDED?
No

ASSISTANCE NEEDED?
No

ACCESSORIES
Finish with a pretty bow or weave a ribbon through your braid for a nice touch.

TRY THIS
Two reverse braids are the basis for the mermaid braid (see pages 62–63), or you could twist your braid up into a bun.

▶ **SEE ALSO**
Dutch braid, pages 44–45
Crowning braid, pages 80–81

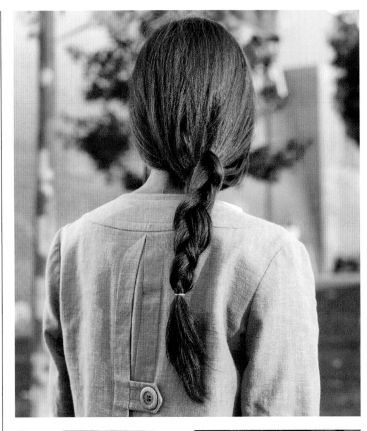

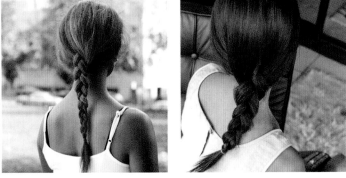

Top: Hairstyling by Christina Butcher, photography by Xiaohan Shen, modeling by Deauvanné.
Bottom left: Hairstyling by Christina Butcher, photography by Xiaohan Shen, modeling by Dorothy Jean Joly.
Bottom right: Hairstyling and photography by Christina Butcher, modeling by Carolyn Mach.

HOW TO GET IT

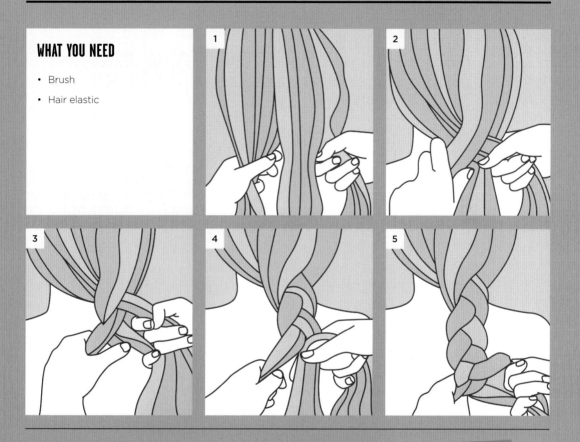

WHAT YOU NEED

- Brush
- Hair elastic

1. Brush your hair to remove any knots and then split your hair into three equal pieces.

2. Take the piece on the left and cross it under the middle piece, into the center. From there, take the piece on the right and cross it under the left (now middle) piece. You'll start to see the braid forming.

3. Take the section now on the left and cross it under and into the middle, and then repeat again, bringing the right under the left (now middle).

4. As you continue down, bring each outer piece under the middle to form the braid.

5. When you're finished, secure the end of the braid with an elastic.

TOP TIP

As with the basic braid, use a small clear elastic to finish, as it won't interfere with the look of the finished upstyle. Stretch the sides of the braid once you have finished to make the braid look fuller and thicker. This will also improve the structure of the braid.

FRENCH BRAID
THE LOOK

The French braid is a classic, timeless hairstyle. It is created by initially following the basic braid technique and then adding in small sections of hair from each side as you continue down the back of your head. The French braid sits close to your head and is a beautiful way to wear your hair up. It looks great in curly, wavy and straight hair types and suits all hair lengths, from shoulder length to extremely long hair.

DIFFICULTY LEVEL
Medium

IDEAL HAIR LENGTH
Medium to long

HAIR EXTENSIONS NEEDED?
No

ASSISTANCE NEEDED?
Yes, but you can do this in your own hair with practice.

ACCESSORIES
Thread ribbon through as you braid to accentuate the structure or use a decorative hair elastic at the end of the braid for a pretty finish.

TRY THIS
Once you've mastered the French braid style, you can move it around to create an infinite number of hairstyles. Try a half braid, diagonal braid, S-shaped braid, or an upside-down braid bun.

▶ **SEE ALSO**
Side French braid, pages 88–89
Upside-down braid bun, pages 136–137

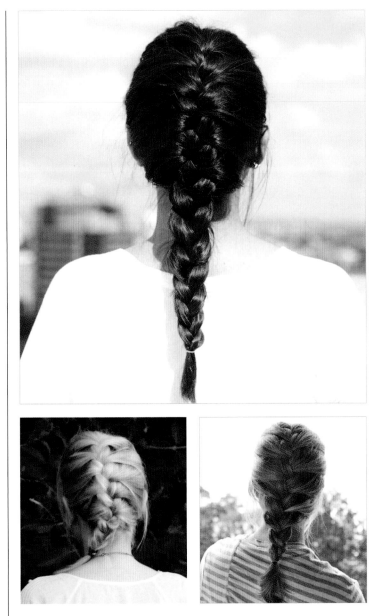

Top: Hairstyling by Christina Butcher, photography by Xiaohan Shen, modeling by Sophia Phan.
Bottom left: Hairstyling, photography, and modeling by Suzy Wimbourne Photography.
Bottom right: Hairstyling and modeling by Christina Butcher, photography by Xiaohan Shen.

HOW TO GET IT

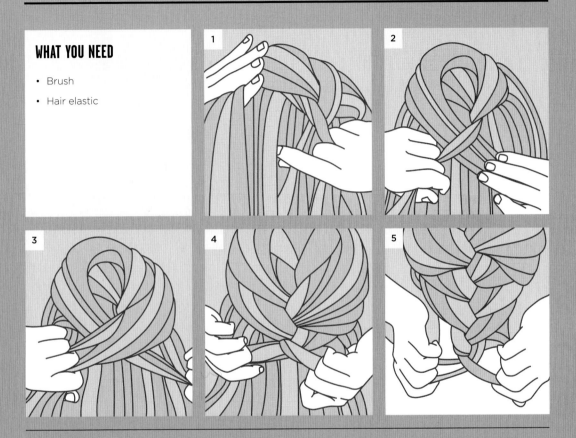

WHAT YOU NEED

- Brush
- Hair elastic

1. Start by taking a section of hair at the top of your head and splitting it into three equal pieces. In the same way that you form a regular braid, bring the left section over the middle and the right over the left (now middle).

2. When you bring your left over the middle again, grab a little extra piece of hair from the left side of your head, combine it with the left section, and bring them into the middle together.

3. Then, on the right side, bring that section over the middle and add in another piece of hair from the right-hand side. This way you keep forming a regular braid but you add in sections of hair as you go.

4. Continue down the back of your head, adding in equal sections of hair to your braid.

5. Once all your hair is added, finish in a basic braid and secure the end with a hair elastic.

TOP TIP

To keep your braid straight, be aware of your dominant hand—if you're right-handed, concentrate on your left hand. Also, look down as you braid. If your head is turned, the braid won't be straight. Make sure you keep the sections that you add in even, and keep the braid taut (but not too tight) as you work.

DUTCH BRAID
THE LOOK

Now that you've practiced doing a basic braid and a French braid, you can move on to the Dutch braid! This style is really just the reverse of a French braid, and is sometimes called an inside-out braid. Instead of bringing pieces over and into the middle, you bring them under and into the middle so that the braid sits proudly on top. This style suits straight hair, but also looks great in curly hair.

DIFFICULTY LEVEL
Medium

IDEAL HAIR LENGTH
Medium to long

HAIR EXTENSIONS NEEDED?
No

ASSISTANCE NEEDED?
Yes, but you can do this in your own hair with practice.

ACCESSORIES
Like with the French braid, you can add ribbons or bows for a sweet look, or add flowers for a bohemian twist.

TRY THIS
This versatile technique can be used in many hairstyles and can be varied to create an infinite number of looks. Try braiding your hair diagonally downward or into an upside-down braid bun (see pages 136–137).

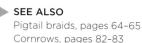
SEE ALSO
Pigtail braids, pages 64–65
Cornrows, pages 82–83

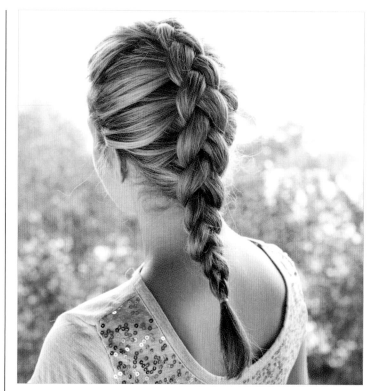

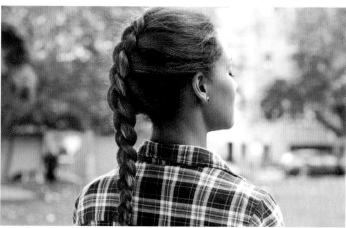

Top: Hairstyling, photography, and modeling by Christina Butcher.
Bottom: Hairstyling by Christina Butcher, photography by Xiaohan Shen, modeling by Dorothy Jean Joly.

HOW TO GET IT

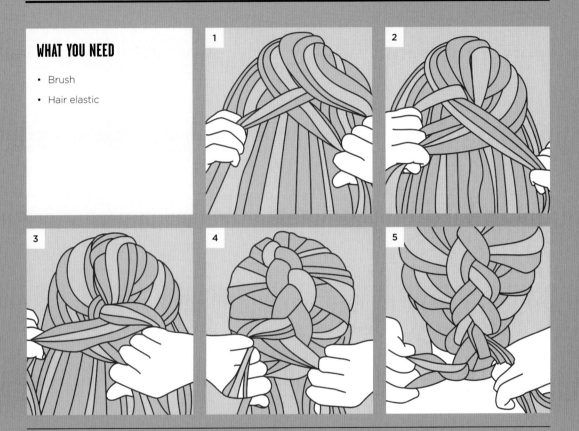

WHAT YOU NEED

- Brush
- Hair elastic

1. Start by taking a section of hair at the top of your head and splitting it into three equal pieces. Begin braiding by taking the left piece under the middle piece and the right piece under the left (now middle) piece.

2. Bring the left piece under the middle again, and add in a small section of hair from the left side.

3. Continue on the right, bringing the right piece under, and adding in a small section of hair from the right-hand side. This way you'll keep forming a reverse braid, but adding in sections of hair underneath as you go.

4. Continue down the back of your head, adding in equal sections of hair to your braid.

5. Once all your hair is added, finish in a reverse braid and secure the end with a hair elastic.

TOP TIP

This braid takes some practice, but you'll actually find it will hold in your hair longer than a French braid because the layers don't need to reach over the top. The Dutch braid looks best when it has been stretched out. You can see the shape better, and it gives the impression of thicker hair.

BRAIDED HEADBAND
THE LOOK

Create the perfect hair accessory using your own hair! Two hidden braids taken from behind your ears cross over the top of your head to form a braided headband. This is a delicate-looking braid, but can be remarkably secure. It adds a countryside feel to your look and so is great for a picnic or spending the day outdoors with friends.

DIFFICULTY LEVEL
Medium

IDEAL HAIR LENGTH
Medium to long

HAIR EXTENSIONS NEEDED?
No

ASSISTANCE NEEDED?
No

ACCESSORIES
Your own hair is the accessory in this hairstyle, so no other adornment is required. However, you could weave flowers or a ribbon through your headband to add an extra dimension to the finished look.

TRY THIS
If you have very long hair, you can just do one braid and cross it over the top of your head. If you have shorter hair, doing two braids makes the headband fuller and the style will look more even.

This style suits straight hair but looks great with wavy or curly hair too. You could also curl the rest of your hair and leave it out or tie it back into a loose bun.

▶ **SEE ALSO**
Heidi braids, pages 74–75
Lace braid, pages 106–107

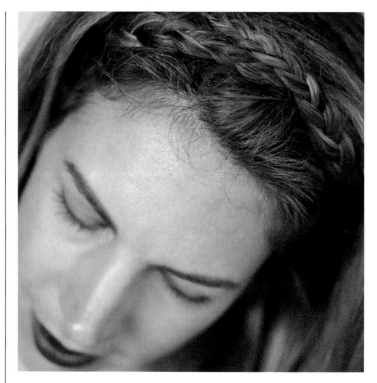

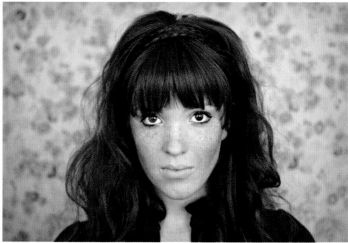

Top: Hairstyling, photography, and modeling by Christina Butcher.
Bottom: Hairstyling, photography, and modeling by Emily M. Meyers/The Freckled Fox.

HOW TO GET IT

WHAT YOU NEED

- Brush
- Hair clip
- 2 small clear hair elastics
- Bobby pins

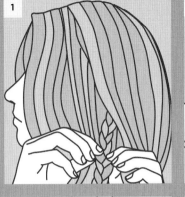

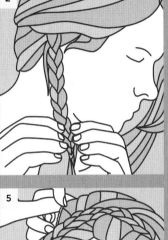

1. Start by brushing all your hair to remove any knots. Clip your hair back and take a 1-inch section of hair from behind your left ear. Braid this section and secure the end with a small clear elastic. Pull at the sides of the braid to loosen it and stretch it out. If you start pulling the braid just above the hair elastic and work back up, you can really enhance the shape of the braid and make your hair look thicker.

2. Repeat on your right side, braiding a 1-inch section of hair behind your right ear. Remember to stretch out your braid.

3–4. Pull one of the braids over your head and into a headband position, and pin in place on top of your hair.

5. Cross the other braid over and pin in place. Tuck the ends of both braids under each other and pin them down to hide them away, and then pin the two braids together for added hold.

TOP TIP

If you have long hair, you may need to braid on only one side to achieve a full headband. Try to braid over the top of your head where the braids will eventually sit; if you start the braids in a downward direction, they won't sit as flat behind your ears.

ANGEL BRAID
THE LOOK

The angel braid is made up of half a French braid, where you only add in hair from one side. Typically, this style is worn along your hairline to keep your hair away from your face. This pretty style can be adapted to sit along the side of your hair or farther back as a braided headband.

DIFFICULTY LEVEL
Medium

IDEAL HAIR LENGTH
Medium to long

HAIR EXTENSIONS NEEDED?
No

ASSISTANCE NEEDED?
No

ACCESSORIES
Your braid acts as a headband in this style, so there's no need for any additional accessories.

TRY THIS
This style looks great in both curly and straight hair. The braid doesn't have to sit at your hairline; try wearing it at the top of your head for a larger headband braid style, or curving it all around into a crowning braid (see pages 80–81).

▶ **SEE ALSO**
Braided headband, pages 46–47
Heart-shaped angel braid, pages 70–71

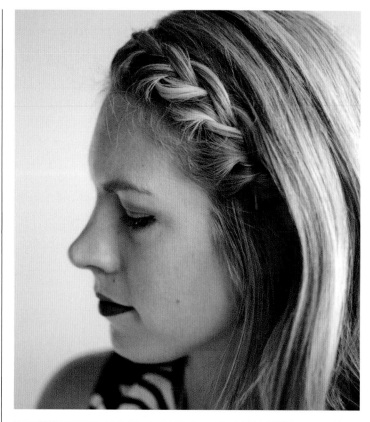

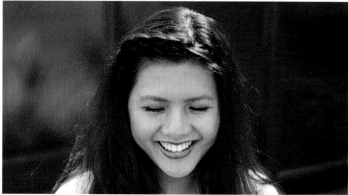

Top: Hairstyling, photography, and modeling by Christina Butcher.
Bottom: Hairstyling by Christina Butcher, photography by Xiaohan Shen, modeling by Sophia Phan.

HOW TO GET IT

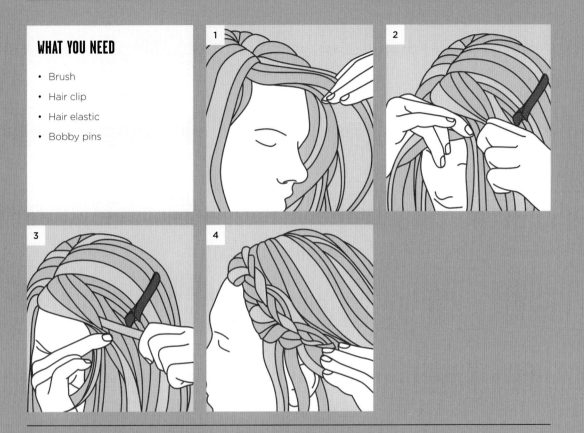

WHAT YOU NEED

- Brush
- Hair clip
- Hair elastic
- Bobby pins

1. Using a brush, make a deep side part on one side of your hair.

2. Section off a 1- to 2-inch section of hair along your hairline. Clip the rest of your hair back out of the way.

3. Split the section in three and start to French braid (see pages 42–43). Instead of adding hair in on both sides of the braid, however, just add in hair from the front. This will add height and create the braid along your hairline, and allow the rest of your hair to sit neatly behind it.

4. Continue to braid down to your ear, adding hair from the front, then finish in a basic braid and secure the end with a hair elastic. Angle the braid back behind your ear and pin in place with bobby pins. Arrange your hair over the top of the end of the braid to hide it.

TOP TIP

If you have bangs, you may end up with layers poking out of the braid. To disguise them, put a bobby pin on the ends of the hair that's sticking out and pin it behind and under the braid to hide them. If you have fine hair, you can lightly tease the top of your hair so that the end of the braid is hidden in your hair.

FISHTAIL BRAID
THE LOOK

This braid is a favorite for long hair because it looks elaborate and difficult but is surprisingly easy to master. The fishtail braid is also referred to as the herringbone or fishbone braid, and is formed by sectioning your hair in two and then crossing over small sections of hair from side to side. It works beautifully in upstyles, as the unique texture adds a stunning twist to buns or chignons.

DIFFICULTY LEVEL
Medium

IDEAL HAIR LENGTH
Long

HAIR EXTENSIONS NEEDED?
No

ASSISTANCE NEEDED?
Yes

ACCESSORIES
The ultimate bohemian look is a messy fishtail braid and a flower crown—nothing too neat or precise with this loose hairstyle.

TRY THIS
Try twisting your fishtail braid into a chignon. The fishtail also adds a unique texture to buns and updos. Stretch the sides of your braid out to create a messy and bohemian look, or make three fishtails and braid them together like a triple braid (see pages 58–59).

▶ **SEE ALSO**
Fishtail crown braids, pages 86–87
Fishtail chignon, pages 160–161

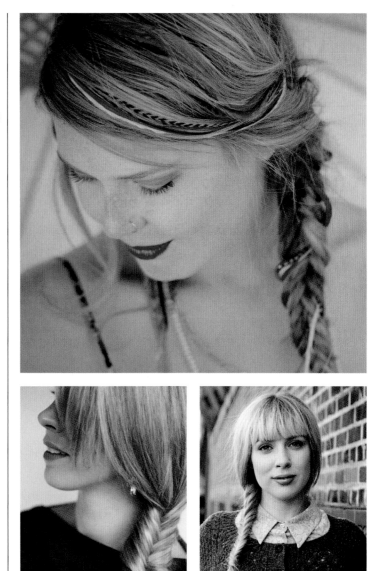

Top: Photograph courtesy of Fine Featherheads. Photography by Kate Broussard, Soulshots Photography.
Bottom left: Hairstyling, photography, and modeling by Christina Butcher.
Bottom right: Photograph courtesy of Brooklyn Tweed. Hairstyling by Karen Schaupeter, photography by Jared Flood, modeling by Hannah Metz.

HOW TO GET IT

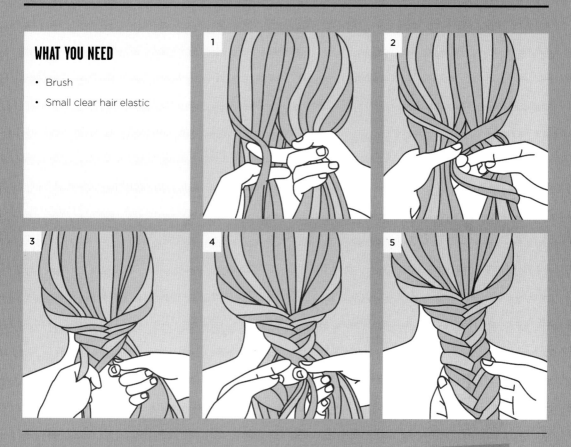

WHAT YOU NEED

- Brush
- Small clear hair elastic

1. Brush your hair to remove any knots. Split your hair into two equal sections. Hold one side in each hand and keep these separate as you braid.

2. Take a small piece of hair from the left side of the left ponytail and cross it over to the right ponytail.

3. Repeat on the right. Take a small piece of hair from the right side of the right ponytail and cross it over to the left ponytail.

4. Repeat this process all the way down your hair. Each time, cross a small piece of hair from one side to the other. As you move down your hair, the pieces will cross over to form the fishtail braid.

5. Secure the end of your fishtail braid with a small clear elastic. Gently pull at the sides of the braid to stretch it out. This will make your hair look thicker and fuller, and emphasize the shape of the braid.

TOP TIP

When you're learning to fishtail braid, it's easier to put your hair up in a ponytail. This is also helpful for keeping your braid in place, especially if you have layers. Doing the fishtail braid while your hair is wet will also make it easier to hold and allow you to be more precise.

FOUR-STRAND BRAID
THE LOOK

Go one up on the basic braid with the four-strand braid. It takes a little practice to master, but it's worth it for the number of compliments you'll receive. Similar to the basic braid, the extra strand woven into this braid creates an intricate woven pattern. Curly and straight hair both look great in this sophisticated updo.

DIFFICULTY LEVEL
Hard

IDEAL HAIR LENGTH
Long

HAIR EXTENSIONS NEEDED?
No

ASSISTANCE NEEDED?
Yes, but you can do this in your own hair with practice.

ACCESSORIES
Finish your braid with a pretty clip, band, or bow. Otherwise, this braid doesn't require any further accessory, as it's the star of this look.

TRY THIS
When braiding your own hair, it's easier to keep track of the pattern and achieve this style as a side braid. Once you are comfortable with this style, try the four-strand French braid (see pages 54–55), which takes this four-strand style to a whole new level.

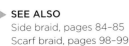

SEE ALSO
Side braid, pages 84–85
Scarf braid, pages 98–99

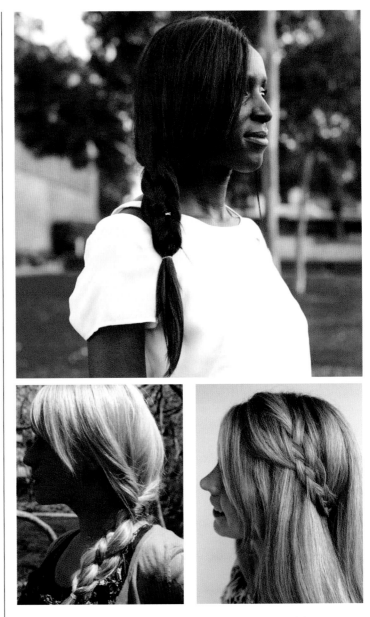

Top: Hairstyling by Christina Butcher, photography by Xiaohan Shen, modeling by Deauvanné.
Bottom left: Hairstyling, photography, and modeling by Abby Smith/Twist Me Pretty.
Bottom right: Hairstyling, photography, and modeling by Christina Butcher.

HOW TO GET IT

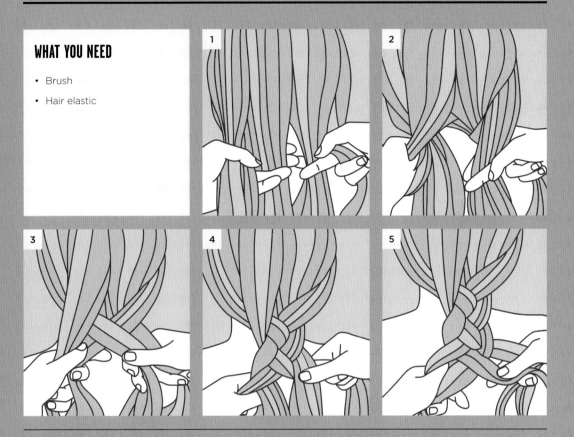

WHAT YOU NEED

- Brush
- Hair elastic

1. Brush your hair to remove any knots before you begin. Divide your hair into two equal sections and split those two sections in half—now you'll have four equal sections.

2. To master this braid, think of each section as a position, numbered 1 to 4 from left to right. Cross 2 over 1 (so right over left) and 4 over 3 (another right over left).

3. Next, cross 1 over 4 into the center (this is left over right with the two new middle sections).

4. Renumber the sections 1 to 4 from left to right and start the process again. Cross 2 over 1 and 4 over 3, then, with the two sections in the center, cross 1 over 4.

5. Keep repeating these steps until you have reached the end of your hair. Secure the end of your braid with a hair elastic.

TOP TIP

It will take a little while to get the hang of this braid, but keep practicing! Remember the pattern of right over left, right over left, then left over right. Saying it aloud while you braid helps you keep track of the next step. Gently stretch out the braid to emphasize the shape and show all four strands.

FOUR-STRAND FRENCH BRAID
THE LOOK

Blow your regular French braid out of the water with the four-strand French braid. This twist on a classic style combines aspects of French and Dutch braids. One side sits out like a Dutch braid, and the other sits flat like a French braid. You'll need to be proficient at the four-strand braid (see pages 52–53) before attempting this French braided version. The complex detail of the two combined braids looks amazing in any type of hair.

DIFFICULTY LEVEL
Hard

IDEAL HAIR LENGTH
Long

HAIR EXTENSIONS NEEDED?
No

ASSISTANCE NEEDED?
Yes

ACCESSORIES
For an elaborate twist, use a small clear elastic to attach a ribbon to a section of hair and include it as the third strand of the braid. Use a ribbon that matches your hair color for a sophisticated look or a bright ribbon for a fun finish.

TRY THIS
Angle your four-strand French braid diagonally down the back of your head for an elegant twist, or twist the end of the braid up and around to form an asymmetrical bun.

▶ **SEE ALSO**
Four-strand braid, pages 52–53
Side French braid, pages 88–89

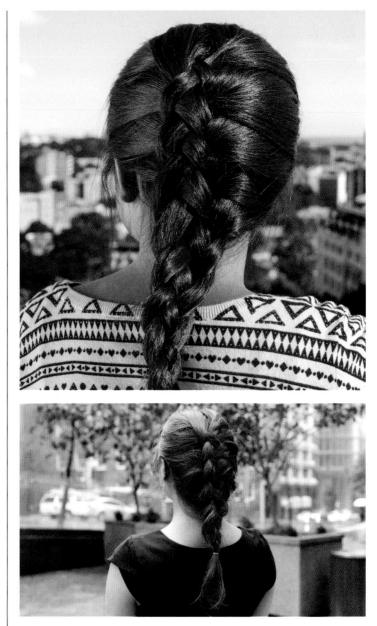

Top: Hairstyling and photography by Christina Butcher, modeling by Adeline Er.
Bottom: Hairstyling by Christina Butcher, photography by Xiaohan Shen, modeling by Ruri Okubo.

HOW TO GET IT

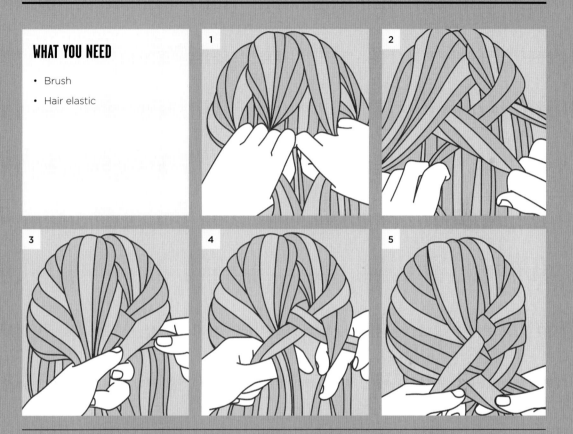

WHAT YOU NEED

- Brush
- Hair elastic

1. Brush your hair to remove any knots before you begin. Take a section of hair at the top of your head and split it into two. Divide those sections again to make four equal sections.

2. To master this braid, think of each section as a position, numbered 1 to 4 from left to right. Cross 2 over 1 (so right over left) and 4 over 3 (another right over left), then 1 crosses over 4 in the center (this is left over right with the two new middle sections).

3. Next, add in small pieces of hair to the sections from the farthest left and right sections. Renumber the sections 1 to 4 from left to right and start the process again. Cross 2 over 1 and 4 over 3, then with the two sections in the center cross 1 over 4.

4. Continue braiding, adding in small pieces of hair to the side sections.

5. Continue down the back of your head. When you run out of hair to add, finish in a four-strand braid and secure the end of your braid with a hair elastic.

TOP TIP

This is a complicated braid and takes practice. Try it out on someone else's hair before attempting it in your own. Don't try to bring in too much hair to positions 1 and 4 each time; a ½-inch or 1-inch section should be enough. Any more than that and the braid will become too big and uneven.

BOW BRAIDS
THE LOOK

Wow your friends with these stunning bow braids. You can integrate the bow braid into almost any style with a French or lace braid technique. This braid is suitable for all hair lengths and layered hair, but works best in straight hair. Make sure to have your answers at the ready though, because everyone will be asking how you did your hair!

DIFFICULTY LEVEL
Hard

IDEAL HAIR LENGTH
Medium to long

HAIR EXTENSIONS NEEDED?
No

ASSISTANCE NEEDED?
Yes

ACCESSORIES
Your hair provides the bows for this style, so there's no need to add any further adornments.

TRY THIS
There are so many ways to use this bow technique in braids and upstyles. Wherever you can do a French braid, you can transform it into bow braids. Simply leave a slim section of hair loose along the edge of your French braid to form the bows. You can try a bow-braided headband, diagonal braid, or bow-braided pigtails.

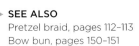 **SEE ALSO**
Pretzel braid, pages 112–113
Bow bun, pages 150–151

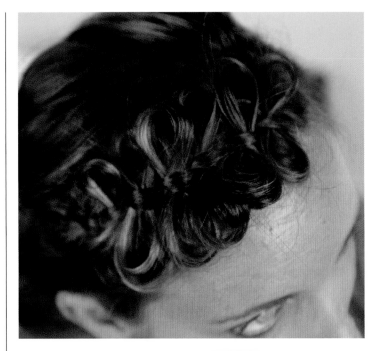

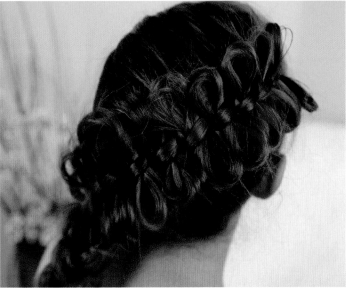

Top and bottom: Hairstyling, photography, and modeling by Mindy McKnight.

56

HOW TO GET IT

WHAT YOU NEED

- Brush
- Fine comb
- Hairspray or pomade
- Hairpin
- Hair elastics

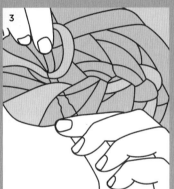

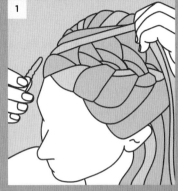

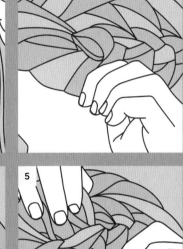

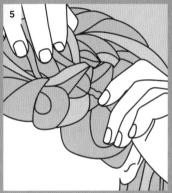

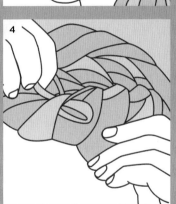

1. Begin by braiding a section of your hair. You can use an angel braid (see pages 48–49) or a French braid (see pages 42–43). Leave a ½-inch section of hair loose, adjacent to your braid, to create the bow.

2. Take a small piece of hair from the ½-inch section and circle it around your finger to create a loop. Place your hairpin, closed end first, through a section of your braid.

3. Thread the loop of hair through the end of your hairpin and take the loop of hair with your left hand while gently pulling the hairpin back through your braid with your right hand.

4. As you bring the hairpin back out of your braid, it will create the other half of the bow. Gently pull the hairpin until you like the look of the second loop and then remove it from your hair. You should now have one completed bow that runs through the braid.

5. Repeat steps 2 to 4 all the way down your braid to create the bows until you run out of hair.

TOP TIP

Depending on the length of your hair, you may have some leftover hair trailing out after making each bow. You can either combine this tail section of hair with the next piece or leave it laying alongside the braid. The next bow loop will cover the loose pieces, so they won't be so obvious.

TRIPLE BRAID
THE LOOK

This easy braid looks so much more complicated than it really is. It's simply three braids woven together to form a single braid. The extra thickness you get from this style will give your hair a lustrous look. It's possible to do this braid in your own hair, though it's easier with some assistance, especially for long hair.

DIFFICULTY LEVEL
Easy

IDEAL HAIR LENGTH
Long

HAIR EXTENSIONS NEEDED?
This style can be achieved in medium-length hair with extensions.

ASSISTANCE NEEDED?
No

ACCESSORIES
This braid doesn't need much adornment, though you could wear flowers in your hair for a bohemian feel.

TRY THIS
You can do this style as a side braid, or try fishtail braids for a beautiful and intricate triple braid. Alternatively, braid only one section out of three to add a pretty detail.

SEE ALSO
Lace braid, pages 106–107
Braided side bun,
pages 158–159

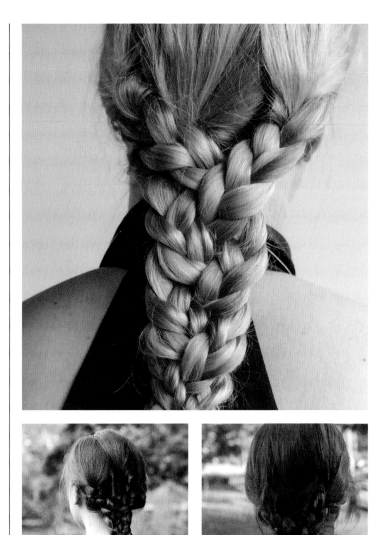

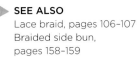
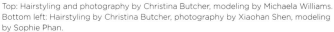

Top: Hairstyling and photography by Christina Butcher, modeling by Michaela Williams.
Bottom left: Hairstyling by Christina Butcher, photography by Xiaohan Shen, modeling by Sophie Phan.
Bottom right: Hairstyling and photography by Christina Butcher, modeling by Nicole Jeyaraj.

HOW TO GET IT

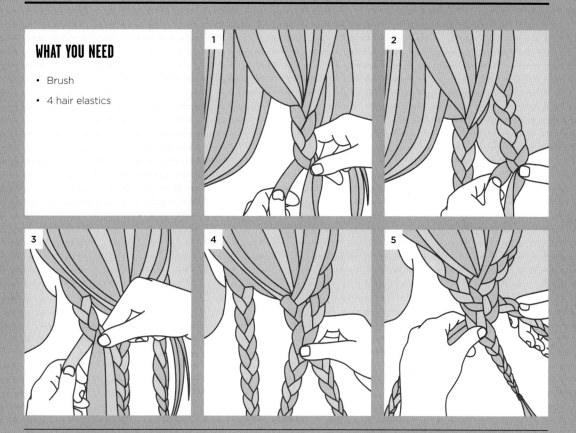

WHAT YOU NEED

- Brush
- 4 hair elastics

1.   Brush your hair to remove any knots and split your hair into three equal sections.

2–3. Braid each section into a basic braid so that you end up with three equal braids. Secure the end of each with an elastic.

4.   Braid the three braids together, again using the basic braid technique.

5.   Secure the ends together with an elastic. That's it!

TOP TIP

Secure each braid with small, clear elastics so that you can't see them. Alternatively, you can remove the elastics from the ends of each braid after you've weaved them together.

BRAIDED KNOT BUNS
THE LOOK

A braided variation on the classic French twist (see pages 130–131), this row of mini braided buns creates a knotted effect down the back of your head. This style looks complicated, but it's not that difficult to do. Working in small, separate sections is key to managing this intriguing style. This updo is made up of four stacked ponytails, one on top of the other at the back of your head, and each bun is independent of each other. You only need to know how to do a basic braid (see pages 38–39) to create this hairstyle. Similar to mini buns (see pages 166–167), this style is more suited to long or thicker hair.

DIFFICULTY LEVEL
Medium

IDEAL HAIR LENGTH
Medium to long

HAIR EXTENSIONS NEEDED?
No

ASSISTANCE NEEDED?
No

ACCESSORIES
The detail in the braided knot buns means that you don't need to add any hair accessories in this style. If you have bangs or layers, use a jeweled clip to pin them back, away from your face.

TRY THIS
If your hair is fine or short, try mini buns instead. Alternatively, customize the style to suit your hair.

▶ **SEE ALSO**
Double bun, pages 140–141
Mini buns, pages 166–167

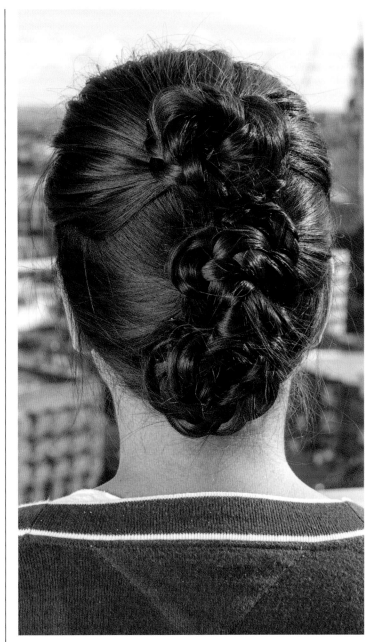

Hairstyling and photography by Christina Butcher, modeling by An Ly.

HOW TO GET IT

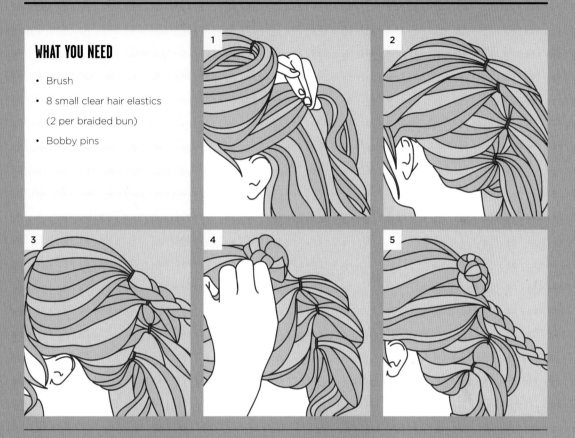

WHAT YOU NEED

- Brush
- 8 small clear hair elastics
  (2 per braided bun)
- Bobby pins

1. Start by brushing all your hair back. You can leave your bangs loose or include them in the style. Take a section of hair running from about your temple back and secure it with a hair elastic.

2. Next, take a section between your temple and your ear and pull it back to make another ponytail section. Secure with a hair elastic. Pull back a third section of hair just level with the back of your ears and make a third ponytail. Gather the rest of your hair into a ponytail directly underneath the other sections you have just made. You should have four ponytails.

3. Braid the top ponytail and secure the end of your braid with an elastic.

4. Wrap the braid around itself and pin in place to make a little bun.

5. Repeat this with the three remaining ponytails to form a vertical row of braided buns.

TOP TIP

Using clear elastics for this style is best, as they don't protrude from the buns and will create a seamless finish. With so many sections, each braid can look a bit thin on its own, so make sure to stretch them out to make them look thicker.

MERMAID BRAID
THE LOOK

The mermaid braid takes your regular side braid and transforms it into something amazing. Best suited to longer hair, the mermaid braid is the perfect summer hairstyle, and is also ideal for a special nighttime date. This stunning braid gives the illusion of being a six-strand braid through the clever use of bobby pins.

DIFFICULTY LEVEL
Medium

IDEAL HAIR LENGTH
Long

HAIR EXTENSIONS NEEDED?
No, but they can be used if you have shorter hair.

ASSISTANCE NEEDED?
No

ACCESSORIES
Apart from the scarf braid variation (see below), it's not necessary to include more hair accessories. Keep the look relaxed and simple, and let the braid shine.

TRY THIS
Try incorporating a scarf into your mermaid braid. Place the scarf around your head and weave it into both reverse braids.

SEE ALSO
Fishtail braid, pages 50–51
Four-strand French braid, pages 54–55

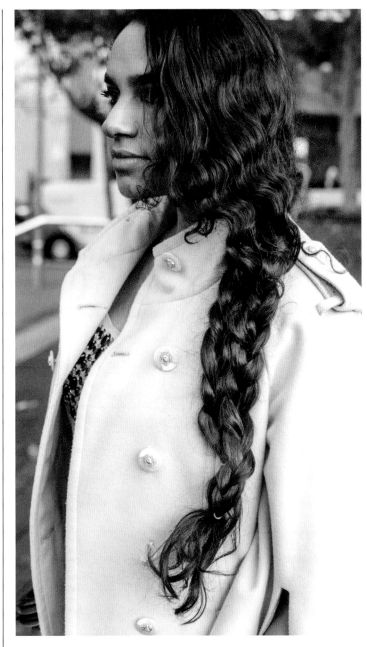

Hairstyling and photography by Christina Butcher, modeling by Tanu Vasu.

HOW TO GET IT

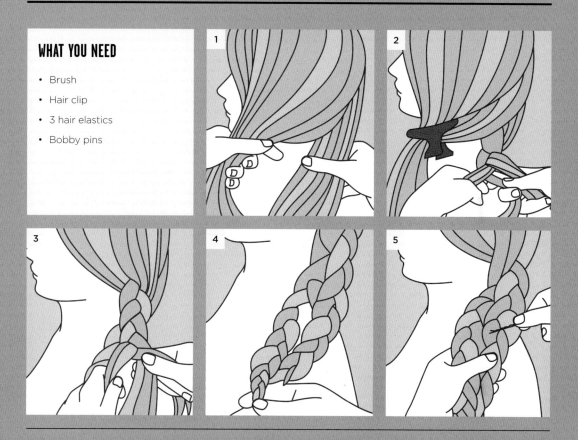

WHAT YOU NEED

- Brush
- Hair clip
- 3 hair elastics
- Bobby pins

1. Brush your hair to remove any knots. Bring your hair over one shoulder and divide into two equal sections.

2. Clip away one section of hair and braid the other section in a reverse braid (see pages 40–41), and secure the end with a hair elastic.

3. Unclip the other section of hair and create another reverse braid. Stretch out the two braids by gently pulling at the sides.

4. Line up the two separate braids so they begin to look like one large braid. Focus on aligning the center of the braids and don't worry if the ends are uneven. It's less important for the outer sides to match, but you do want to make the center appear to be one single braid.

5. Use bobby pins to connect the center of the two braids together, edge to edge. Angle your pins through both braids and push them vertically at the end to secure them. You'll need to place your pins about every 1 or 1 1/2 inches. Join both braids together with a hair elastic.

TOP TIP

You can remove the hair elastics from the two braids and just use one to combine them together. If you use clear elastics, this isn't important, as they are more inconspicuous. Don't worry about making the two reverse braids too neat; the style will look better messy.

PIGTAIL BRAIDS
THE LOOK

Frame your face with these sweet pigtails, which begin with a Dutch braid at the top (see page 44) and at ear level combine with the rest of your hair to finish in a basic braid. By stretching out the braids, you'll emphasize their shape. To keep the look modern, leave the braids slightly messy and a little softer, with some loose layers at the front.

DIFFICULTY LEVEL
Medium

IDEAL HAIR LENGTH
Medium to long

HAIR EXTENSIONS NEEDED?
No

ASSISTANCE NEEDED?
No

ACCESSORIES
Keep this hairstyle simple and modern by leaving off the bows and ribbons. Less is more when you're wearing pigtails.

TRY THIS
If pigtails aren't your thing, you can easily convert this daytime hairstyle into a more sophisticated look by pinning them up. Fold and cross the pigtails over and pin them at the nape of your neck for an elegant upstyle.

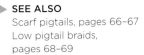

SEE ALSO
Scarf pigtails, pages 66–67
Low pigtail braids, pages 68–69

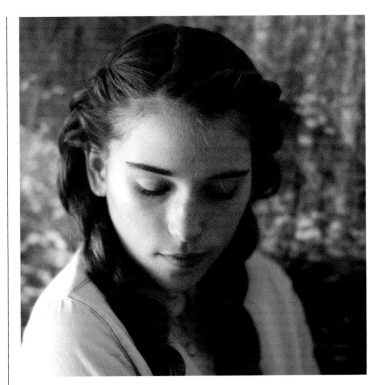

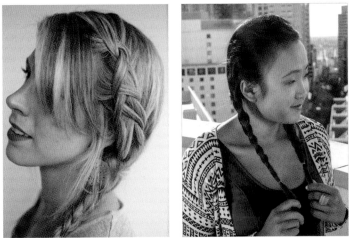

Top: Hairstyling, photography, and modeling by Alison Titus.
Bottom left: Hairstyling, photography, and modeling by Christina Butcher.
Bottom right: Hairstyling and photography by Christina Butcher, modeling by Adeline Er.

HOW TO GET IT

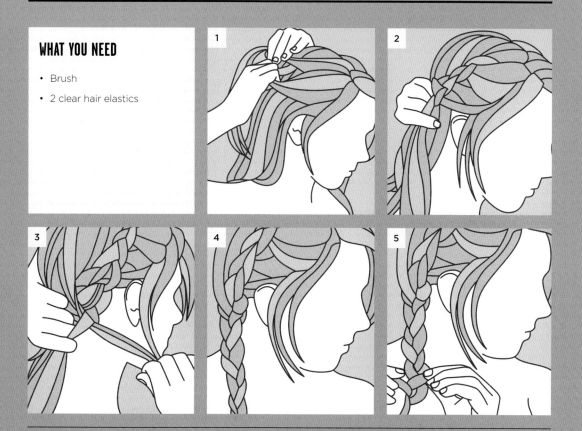

WHAT YOU NEED

- Brush
- 2 clear hair elastics

1. Loosely split your hair down the middle into two equal bunches.

2. Take a 1-inch section of hair near your part and start a Dutch braid (see pages 44–45) along your hairline.

3. Continue down to your ear, adding in hair from both sides as you braid.

4. Once you pass your ear, add in the rest of your hair and continue in a regular braid to finish the pigtail. Use a clear elastic to secure the end of the braid.

5. Repeat on the other side. When you're done, stretch out each braid to emphasize their shape.

TOP TIP

To create a seamless transition from the Dutch braid to the regular braid at your ear, take the Dutch braid as one section. Split the rest of your hair in two to make up the other two sections of the braid. If you have bangs, you can leave them loose or add them into the Dutch braid.

SCARF PIGTAILS
THE LOOK

In this hairstyle a scarf becomes a special feature. It sits like a headband across the top of your head and is then used as a section in each pigtail braid, helping to make your hair look thicker. Because the scarf can add color to your hair, it can be used to complement whatever you're wearing. Straight or curly hair looks great in this style.

DIFFICULTY LEVEL
Medium

IDEAL HAIR LENGTH
Medium to long

HAIR EXTENSIONS NEEDED?
No

ASSISTANCE NEEDED?
No

ACCESSORIES
A large rectangular scarf is easy to work into this style, but if you have a square scarf, simply fold it diagonally until you get a 2-inch-wide strip. The choice of scarf will transform the look of this braid. Pick a neutral tone for an elegant style or a bright, colorful scarf for a fun, flirty look.

TRY THIS
Pigtails not your thing? This style looks gorgeous with the braids pinned up at the nape of your neck. Fold the braid up, tucking the ends under, and pin in place. Pin the second braid over the top of the first for a beautiful braided updo.

SEE ALSO
Low pigtail braids, pages 68–69
Scarf braid, pages 98–99

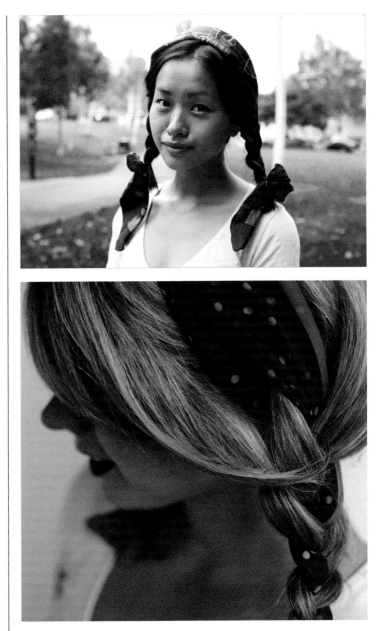

Top: Hairstyling by Christina Butcher, photography by Xiaohan Shen, modeling by Jessica Tran.
Bottom: Hairstyling, photography, and modeling by Christina Butcher.

HOW TO GET IT

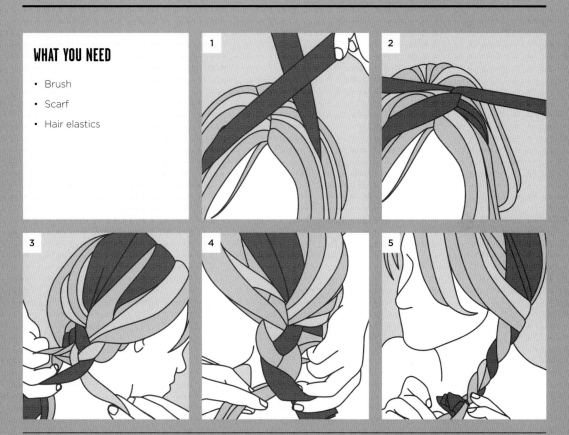

WHAT YOU NEED

- Brush
- Scarf
- Hair elastics

1. Brush and loosely part your hair. Place the scarf around the back of your neck, and bring it up like a headband.

2. Twist the ends of the scarf around each other to form a turban-style knot.

3. Bring the ends of your scarf down on either side and make sure they're about the same length as your hair. Secure one side of your hair and one end of the scarf with a hair elastic (this helps keep the tension in the scarf and stops the knot from moving as you braid the other side).

4. The scarf will form one of the three sections of the regular braid. Split the rest of your hair in two and use the scarf as the center section, then just weave the two hair sections and the scarf into a regular braid and secure with a clear elastic.

5. Repeat on the other side.

TOP TIP

If your hair is very long, you may not need to put the scarf around the back of your head to do the first headband piece. Instead, you could place the scarf over your head, trailing the ends down on either side as part of the pigtails. You want the ends of the scarf to be about level with the ends of your hair.

LOW PIGTAIL BRAIDS
THE LOOK

Channel your inner hippy with these relaxed low pigtails. This casual hairstyle is ideal for a carefree summer's day. A loose center part, with slightly messy, textured hair, leads to two low pigtail braids that let your hair down in the best possible way. Great for straight or curly hair, you're ready to skip to Coachella with this bohemian upstyle.

DIFFICULTY LEVEL
Easy

IDEAL HAIR LENGTH
Medium to long

HAIR EXTENSIONS NEEDED?
No, but they can be used in short hair.

ASSISTANCE NEEDED?
No

ACCESSORIES
Embrace your inner bohemian and wear your low pigtails with a flower crown. Weave daisies through your pigtails for the perfect summer festival hairstyle. Tie red bows at the ends of your low pigtails for a cute Bavarian look.

TRY THIS
For an even more carefree look, tie your hair into two ponytails and encourage natural texture with a sea salt spray.

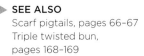

SEE ALSO
Scarf pigtails, pages 66–67
Triple twisted bun, pages 168–169

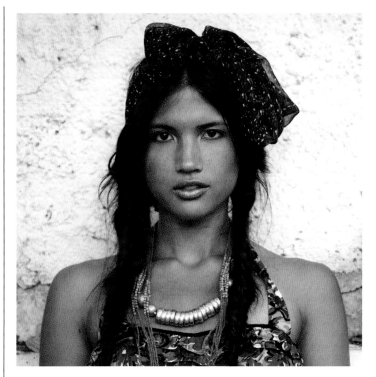

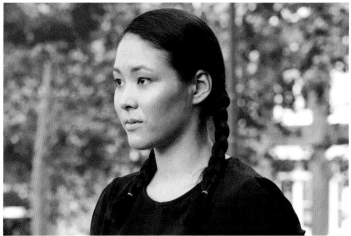

Top: Hairstyling by Cristi Cagle, photography by Lou Mora, makeup by Jennifer Fiamengo.
Bottom: Hairstyling by Christina Butcher, photography by Xiaohan Shen, modeling by Tash Williams.

HOW TO GET IT

WHAT YOU NEED

- Brush
- Hair clip (optional)
- 2 hair elastics

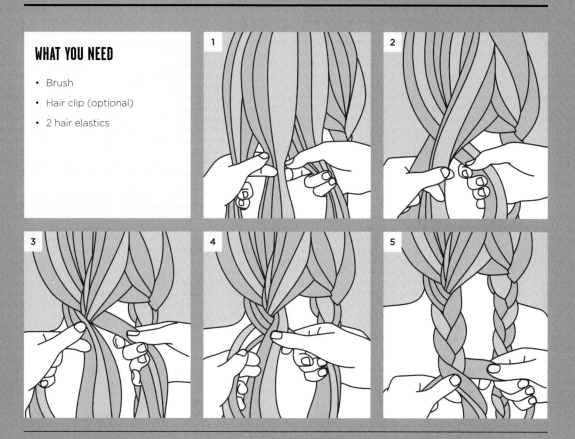

1–4. Brush your hair to remove any knots, but don't brush too much—you don't need to start with perfect hair for this style. Make a rough center part with your fingers. If you find it easier, clip one side out of the way with your hair clip. Finger-tease your hair and form a low basic braid. Secure the end of your braid with a hair elastic.

5. Repeat on the other side.

TOP TIP

To give this style a more modern feel, don't make it look too perfect. Create the part with your fingers and lightly muss up your hair or backcomb with your fingers before starting the braid to give it a more lived-in, contemporary feel.

HEART-SHAPED ANGEL BRAID
THE LOOK

Love is in the hair! You can actually wear your heart in your hair with this romantic braided hairstyle. This look uses a technique similar to the angel braid to create a heart-shaped outline. Although it might seem impossible, this style isn't as hard to master as you'd think!

DIFFICULTY LEVEL
Medium

IDEAL HAIR LENGTH
Medium to long

HAIR EXTENSIONS NEEDED?
No

ASSISTANCE NEEDED?
Yes, but you can do this in your own hair with practice.

ACCESSORIES
Add a red or pink ribbon at the bottom of the heart for an extra-sweet finish.

TRY THIS
This heart stands out clearly on straight hair but you can also curl the ends of your hair for a more romantic hairstyle. Instead of finishing in a half-up style, incorporate your heart-shaped angel braid into a low ponytail.

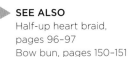
SEE ALSO
Half-up heart braid, pages 96–97
Bow bun, pages 150–151

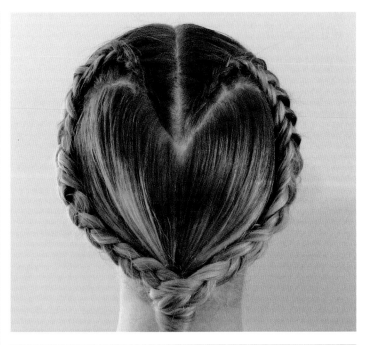

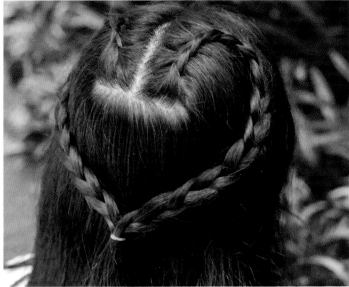

Top: Hairstyling, photography, and modeling by Jemma Grace.
Bottom: Hairstyling and photography by Christina Butcher, modeling by Riko Ishihata.

HOW TO GET IT

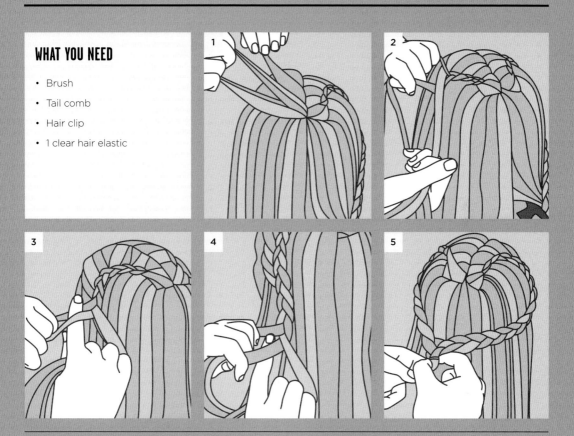

WHAT YOU NEED

- Brush
- Tail comb
- Hair clip
- 1 clear hair elastic

1. Brush your hair and create a deep center part with your tail comb. Use your hair clip to keep half your hair away while you do the first braid.

2. Make a horizontal part at the crown, running from your center part to your ear. Pick up a section of hair at the crown and split into three.

3. Begin your angel braid (see pages 48–49), angling it toward your face, only adding in hair on the outer side of the braid. After you have added about three pieces to the braid, turn the braid by angling it toward your ear to create the rounded top of the heart.

4. Continue braiding the heart shape, only adding in hair from the front until you reach the ear. At this point, stop adding hair and continue with a basic braid until you reach the middle of your head at your neckline. Secure with a hair elastic. Release the clip from the other side and repeat the angel braid on the other side to match the first.

5. Connect the two braids at the back of your head with the clear elastic to form the bottom of the heart.

TOP TIP

To keep the heart shape as even as possible, only add in small sections to your braid. Keep the braids quite tight so that you can see where it's going and make adjustments as you go.

SHORT HAIR BRAID
THE LOOK

You really don't need long hair to be able to wear a braid. Lace braids (see pages 106–107) can also work in short hair, and this Dutch-style braid is perfect for shorter hair. The braid runs around your hairline and finishes behind your ear. The rest of your hair can be twisted into a low updo or left out. As long as your hair is at least 3 inches long, you can do this braid. Curly hair looks awesome in this style.

DIFFICULTY LEVEL
Medium

IDEAL HAIR LENGTH
Short

HAIR EXTENSIONS NEEDED?
No

ASSISTANCE NEEDED?
No

ACCESSORIES
You can use a flower corsage or jeweled pin in your hair to accent this hairstyle, but this is a personal choice. The braids add unique detail to a shorter style, so extra accessories are really not necessary.

TRY THIS
Depending on the length and thickness of your hair, you could do two Dutch braids next to each other to create a more distinctive braided look.

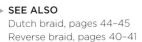
SEE ALSO
Dutch braid, pages 44–45
Reverse braid, pages 40–41

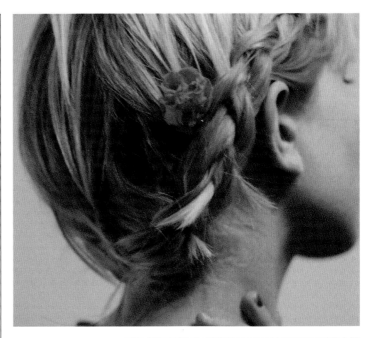

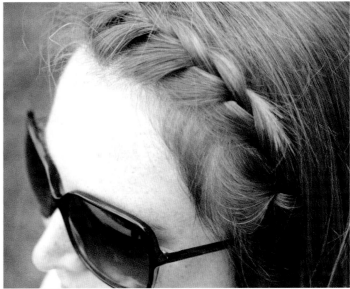

Top: Hairstyling, photography, and modeling by Suzy Wimbourne Photography.
Bottom: Hairstyling and photography by Christina Butcher, modeling by Barbara Rainbird.

HOW TO GET IT

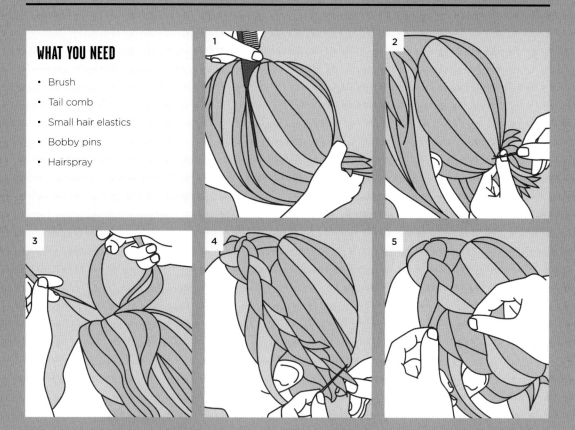

WHAT YOU NEED

- Brush
- Tail comb
- Small hair elastics
- Bobby pins
- Hairspray

1. Brush your hair to remove any knots. Use a tail comb to create a part across the top of your head from ear to ear. Brush the front section forward.

2. Gather the rest of your hair in a small elastic at the back. Depending on the length of your hair, twist and pin the back of your hair into a little bun and secure with bobby pins.

3. Next, take a section of hair at the front and split it into three. Make a Dutch braid (see pages 44–45) following your hairline around to your bun at the back.

4. Pin the ends of your braid into your bun with bobby pins.

5. Pull at the edges of your braid to emphasize the shape. Pin any loose pieces, but leave a few loose layers of hair around your face. Use hairspray to finish the style so that it holds in your hair.

TOP TIP

To give your hair some texture, volume, and body, curl your hair before you begin using a 1-inch barrel curling iron. A volumizing mousse or pomade will also aid in giving your hair more texture.

HEIDI BRAIDS
THE LOOK

Leave Heidi behind frolicking in the Swiss Alpine meadows! The sweet, girlish charm of this braided style is easily updated to a modern, wearable look. Best in long hair, Heidi braids are formed by making low pigtails and pinning the braids up and over to form a kind of headband. Pulling at the sides of the braids encourages your hair's natural texture and makes this hairstyle look even more modern.

DIFFICULTY LEVEL
Medium

IDEAL HAIR LENGTH
Long

HAIR EXTENSIONS NEEDED?
No

ASSISTANCE NEEDED?
No

ACCESSORIES
Heidi braids look beautiful accessorized with a scarf or ribbon. To do this, incorporate a scarf as one section of the braid and connect it across the back of your head to the other braid. You can also weave a ribbon through the finished style for added color.

TRY THIS
A center part is the classic look for this braid, but try varying the style with a side part or zigzag part. Instead of a regular braid, try a fishtail braid to create an intricate, on-trend look.

SEE ALSO
Braided headband, pages 46–47
Scarf braid, pages 98–99

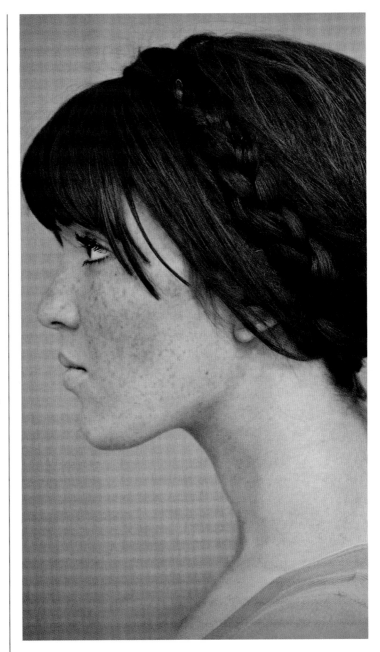

Hairstyling, photography, and modeling by Emily M. Meyers/The Freckled Fox.

HOW TO GET IT

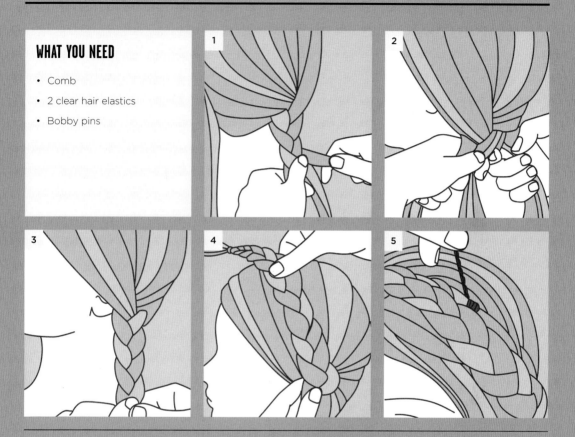

WHAT YOU NEED

- Comb
- 2 clear hair elastics
- Bobby pins

1. Using a comb, part your hair down the center from your forehead to the nape of your neck to create two equal sections.

2. Take the first section, split it into three equal sections, and make a basic braid, starting just behind your ear. Secure the end of your braid with a clear elastic.

3. Repeat, braiding the section on the other side.

4. Holding the start of your braid with one hand, pull the end of one braid up and over the top of your head. Pin in place with bobby pins.

5. Repeat with the second braid. Tuck the ends of both braids underneath each other, and secure with bobby pins. Place a couple of pins through both braids to join them together, and also pin the to the hair below so the style holds.

TOP TIP

When you are braiding, pull your hair down and slightly forward to keep it taut. This way, when you pull the braids up and over your head, you won't have too much loose hair at the back. Don't forget the braids are going up and over the top of your head, not down like most braids.

FIGURE-8 BRAID
THE LOOK

This intricate braid is sometimes known as an infinity braid because the figure-8 pattern looks like the infinity symbol. To create this style, you'll horizontally wrap a small piece of hair in and around two sections of hair, forming the infinity "8" shape. In line with its design, the number of places you can wear this sleek, distinctive braid are limitless!

DIFFICULTY LEVEL
Medium

IDEAL HAIR LENGTH
Long

HAIR EXTENSIONS NEEDED?
No

ASSISTANCE NEEDED?
Yes

ACCESSORIES
To add some color, try tying a ribbon around one of the winding sections and weaving it through the braid. A simple bow or clip at the end of the braid is also a nice touch.

TRY THIS
This unique braid can be worn in a half-up style or as a side braid, and you can incorporate this braid in your hair wherever you would wear a fishtail braid. It also creates beautiful texture when twisted up into a bun.

▶ **SEE ALSO**
Fishtail braid, pages 50–51
Fishtail crown braids, pages 86–87

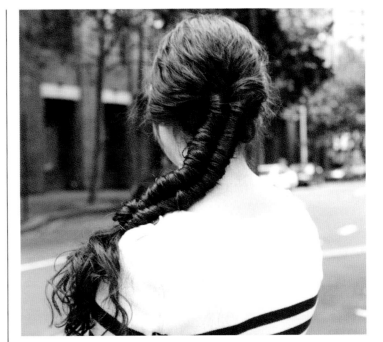

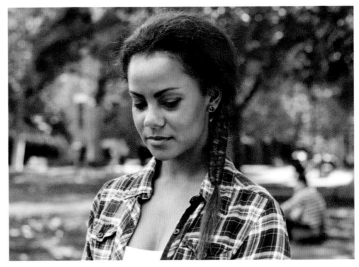

Top: Hairstyling by Christina Butcher, photography by Xiaohan Shen, modeling by Monica Bowerman .
Bottom: Hairstyling by Christina Butcher, photography by Xiaohan Shen, modeling by Dorothy Jean Joly.

HOW TO GET IT

WHAT YOU NEED

- Brush or comb
- Hair elastic

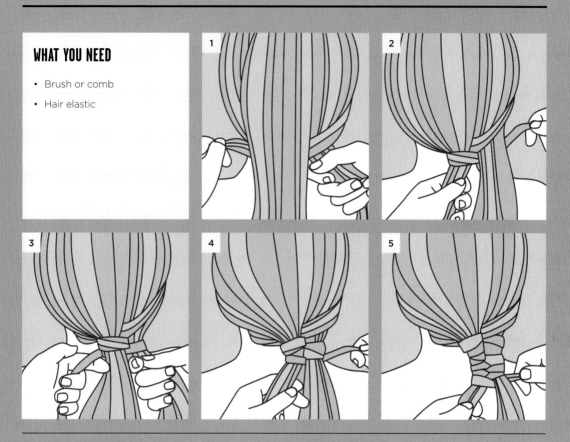

1. Brush your hair to remove any knots. Split your hair into two equal sections. Take a small piece of hair from the outside of the right section and bring it over the right section and under the left section.

2. Next, bring the piece of hair over the left section and under the right section.

3. Continue in a figure-8 pattern, wrapping the piece of hair around the two sections.

4. When you start to run out of hair, add in another small piece of hair from the side and continue in the figure-8 shape.

5. Continue all the way down your hair and secure the end with an elastic.

TOP TIP

It's important to keep the looping figure-8 pattern tight as you braid. Keep the tension in the weaving piece of hair—this will keep the shape of the braid consistent.

GRECIAN BRAID
THE LOOK

Inspired by classics from the silver screen, this beautiful braid pays tribute to the elegance and simplicity of the ancient Greeks. You'll form this hairstyle by French braiding in a ring following your hairline, beginning at your right ear and braiding over your forehead, following your hairline until you run out of hair. Wear this braid in the sunshine—it's perfect for picnics, the beach, festivals . . . and toga parties!

DIFFICULTY LEVEL
Hard

IDEAL HAIR LENGTH
Medium to long

HAIR EXTENSIONS NEEDED?
No

ASSISTANCE NEEDED?
Yes, but you can do this in your own hair with practice.

ACCESSORIES
This eye-catching braid doesn't need any additional hair accessories, but focus on other items, such as earrings or a necklace, to complement your hair.

TRY THIS
If your hair is very long, you can complete this look by winding the braid into a bun and pinning it at the back of your head. If you have shorter hair, keep the braid nearer your crown and you should be able to go full circle with the hair you have. This should also help the braid stay secure.

▶ **SEE ALSO**
French braid, pages 42–43
Crowning braid, pages 80–81

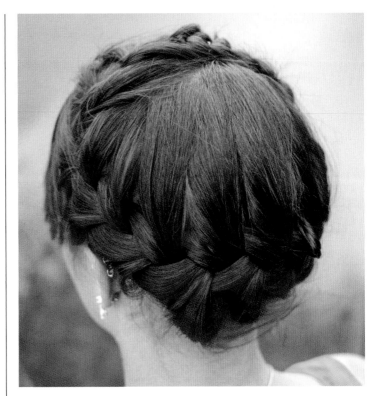

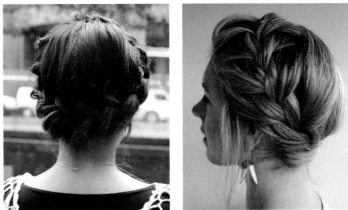

Top: Hairstyling and photography by Christina Butcher, modeling by Elly Hanson.
Bottom left: Hairstyling by Christina Butcher, photography by Xiaohan Shen, modeling by Teru Morihira.
Bottom right: Hairstyling, photography, and modeling by Christina Butcher.

HOW TO GET IT

WHAT YOU NEED

- Brush or comb
- Hair elastic
- Bobby pins and/or hairpins

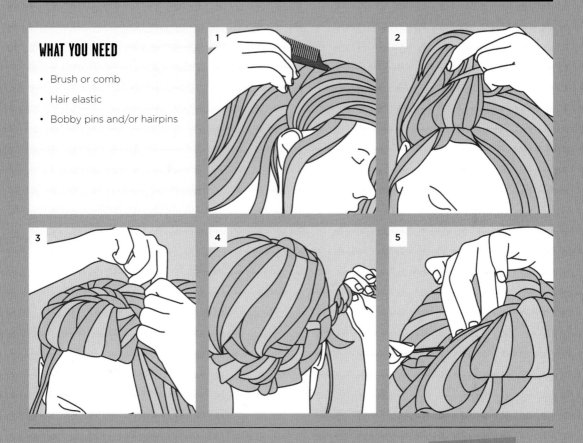

1. Take a section of hair above your right ear and split it into three.

2. Begin to French braid (see pages 42–43), adding in hair from both your hairline and from the crown behind. If you're left-handed, start at the top of your left ear and work round in the opposite direction to the instructions here. Using your stronger hand will help you make a neater braid.

3. Braid across your forehead and behind your left ear. As you reach the back of your left ear, keep following your hands around, keeping tension in the braid. Follow your hairline around the back of your head. By the time you reach the bottom right-hand side of your neck, you'll have added in all your hair.

4. Finish in a regular braid and secure with a small clear elastic.

5. Stretch out the braid, tuck the end under the start of the braid behind your right ear, and pin in place with bobby pins.

TOP TIP

If you like to have a little bit of height in the hair around your face, sit this braid about an inch back from your hairline. You can then gently stretch the braid out to adjust how your hair sits at the front. Use hairpins to pin the braid in place if you have long or thick hair.

CROWNING BRAID
THE LOOK

A pretty twist on a half-up hairstyle, crowning braids are formed by crossing over two braids at the back of your head. This style is an excellent look for weddings, whether you're part of the bridal party or a guest. Because all the detail is at the back, a veil or half veil looks beautiful pinned into the braids. This half-up, half-down style looks best with loose layers at the front and bangs left long and unstyled.

DIFFICULTY LEVEL
Medium

IDEAL HAIR LENGTH
Medium to long

HAIR EXTENSIONS NEEDED?
No

ASSISTANCE NEEDED?
No

ACCESSORIES
For a colorful twist, weave a fine ribbon through the finished braids so that it runs in and out of the inner edges. You can also add a headband or use a jeweled clip to pin back your bangs.

TRY THIS
Different techniques can add stunning detail to this simple style. Try other types of braids, such as the fishtail braid (see pages 50–51), the uneven braid (see pages 90–91), or the slide-up braid (see pages 100–101).

▶ **SEE ALSO**
Fishtail crown braids, pages 86–87
Half-up heart braid, pages 96–97

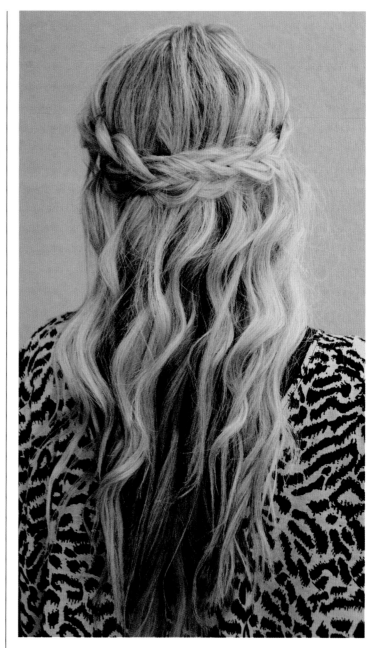

Hairstyling, photography, and modeling by Abby Smith/Twist Me Pretty.

HOW TO GET IT

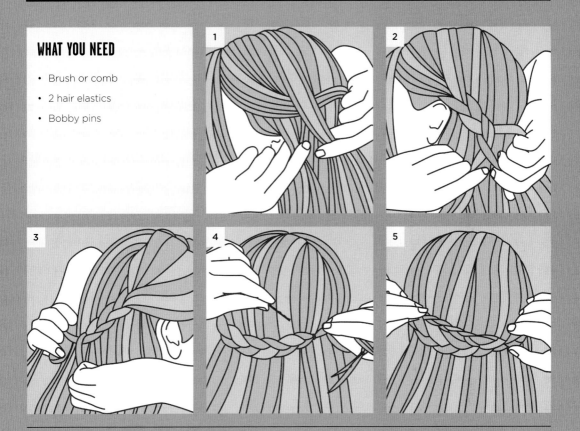

WHAT YOU NEED

- Brush or comb
- 2 hair elastics
- Bobby pins

1. Brush or comb your hair and part it down the middle. Gather two large sections of hair on each side of your face above your ears. Split one of the sections in three.

2. Begin braiding. Start loosely at the top, and angle your braid back. This way the braid will sit in the direction that you want the finished style to be. Secure the end of the braid with an elastic.

3. Repeat on the opposite side, making a braid above your other ear.

4. Cross the first braid behind your head and pin in place with bobby pins, making sure to tuck in the ends.

5. Cross the second braid behind your head and pin it level with the first braid, tucking the ends in underneath.

TOP TIP

If your braid is quite long, you can fold it in half and tuck the ends in behind the braid. To keep the two braids neat and close together as they cross, push pins in between the two braids so that they are connected and fixed down more securely. Pull the sides of the braids out to give them shape and body.

CORNROWS
THE LOOK

Cornrows are a traditional African hairstyle and braiding technique. These microbraids might be time-consuming, but they have a lot of impact and can last longer than other braided hairstyles. If you have the time, go for a full head of cornrows, or opt to integrate them into other hairstyles as an accent. Depending on how you wear them, cornrows look great for a big night out or a day in town with friends, and are especially great for the beach.

DIFFICULTY LEVEL
Medium to hard

IDEAL HAIR LENGTH
Any

HAIR EXTENSIONS NEEDED?
No

ASSISTANCE NEEDED?
Yes

ACCESSORIES
Cornrows are traditionally decorated with beads and shells.

TRY THIS
There are so many ways to incorporate cornrows into your favorite hairstyle. Try wearing them on the side to create a sweeping part, almost like an undercut. Depending on your skill level and patience, you can create patterns with your cornrows by zigzagging and deviating the braids as you go.

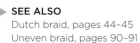
SEE ALSO
Dutch braid, pages 44–45
Uneven braid, pages 90–91

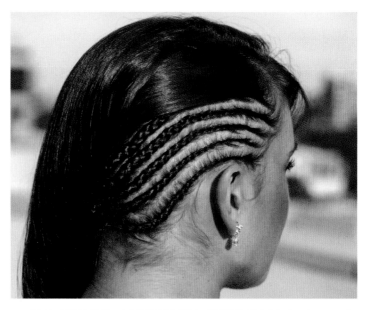

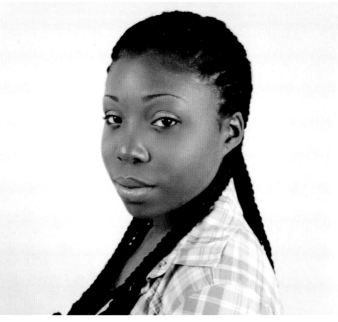

Top: Hairstyling and photography by Christina Butcher, modeling by Elly Hanson.
Bottom: Hairstyling, photography and modeling by Breanna Rutter/How To Black Hair LLC.

HOW TO GET IT

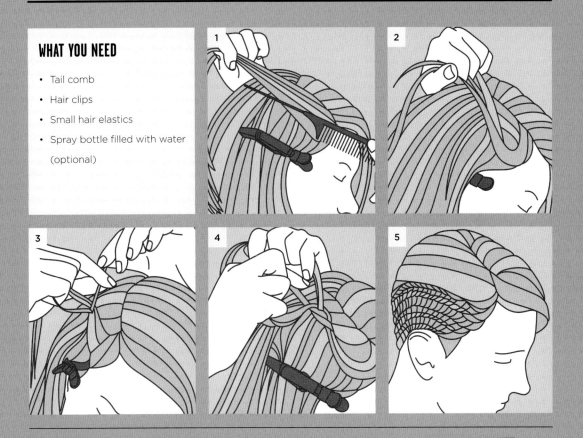

WHAT YOU NEED

- Tail comb
- Hair clips
- Small hair elastics
- Spray bottle filled with water (optional)

1. Use your tail comb to create a neat section for your cornrow braid. Clip the rest of your hair out of the way while you braid.

2. Split the start of the section in three and start to create a Dutch braid (see pages 44-45).

3. Add in small sections as you braid, always bringing the hair in from underneath.

4. When you have run out of hair, finish in a regular braid and secure the end with a small hair elastic.

5. Repeat over the rest of your head, making sure you take equal sections so that your cornrows are the same size.

TOP TIP

It takes time to get these braids to sit correctly. If you start with a larger braid and keep practicing, you will eventually master the technique. It helps to make neat sections, and to clip away the rest of your hair while you're working. Use water in a spray bottle to dampen your hair as you work.

SIDE BRAID
THE LOOK

For a casual yet confident look, try out a side braid. The relaxed feel of this braid works well for a casual night out and can also be dressed up for date night or a day at the office. Because side braids are so versatile and one of the easiest ways to wear your hair, this is an essential style to master.

DIFFICULTY LEVEL
Easy

IDEAL HAIR LENGTH
Long

HAIR EXTENSIONS NEEDED?
No

ASSISTANCE NEEDED?
No

ACCESSORIES
This style is best left simple, so choose jewelry that fits with your long braid. If you want to add something to the style, weave fresh flowers through your braid, or finish with a loose bow.

TRY THIS
A fishtail or mermaid braid would look great in this loose, relaxed style, and would add a bohemian edge.

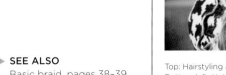

SEE ALSO
Basic braid, pages 38–39
Mermaid braid, pages 62–63

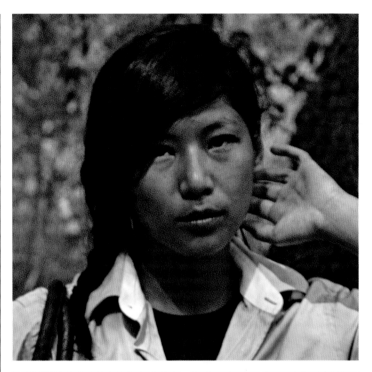

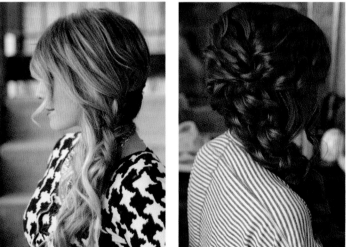

Top: Hairstyling and modeling by Lesly Lotha/Lazymanxcat, photography by Urvashi Das.
Bottom left: Hairstyling, photography and modelling by Abby Smith/Twist Me Pretty.
Bottom right: Hairstyling and photography by Marie-Pierre Sander.

HOW TO GET IT

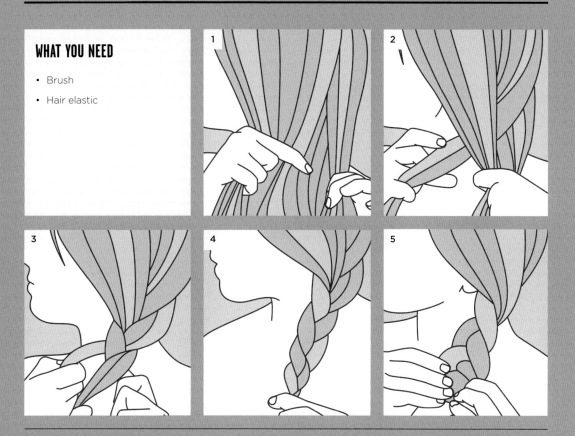

WHAT YOU NEED

- Brush
- Hair elastic

1. Brush your hair to remove any knots before you begin.

2. Make a deep side part on one side of your head and gather a large section of your hair to the other side, over your shoulder.

3. Split this large section of hair into three equal sections and form a basic braid, crossing the right section over the middle and the left section over the right.

4. Continue braiding all of your hair down over your shoulder and secure the end with an elastic.

5. Stretch the sides of your braid to make it appear fuller and so that it sits forward over your shoulder.

TOP TIP

Keep this hairstyle loose for a soft, relaxed look. Start the braid low down and let any shorter layers fall into the start of the braid. Pull at the edges of the braid to give your hair a full-bodied and casual look.

FISHTAIL CROWN BRAIDS
THE LOOK

The gorgeous half crown of braids in this style is created by connecting two fishtail braids from your temples to the back of your head. This pretty half-up braid can be worn as an everyday hairstyle and is perfect for a beach wedding. Half-crown braids are also great for keeping your hair out of your eyes when wearing your hair down. This style works well in straight or curly hair.

DIFFICULTY LEVEL
Medium

IDEAL HAIR LENGTH
Medium to long

HAIR EXTENSIONS NEEDED?
No

ASSISTANCE NEEDED?
Yes

ACCESSORIES
Weave flowers through the braid to create a flower crown or adorn the back of the braid with a bow for a pretty finish.

TRY THIS
If you haven't mastered the fishtail braid, you can use the regular braid technique instead to achieve a similar half-crown style.

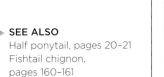
SEE ALSO
Half ponytail, pages 20–21
Fishtail chignon, pages 160–161

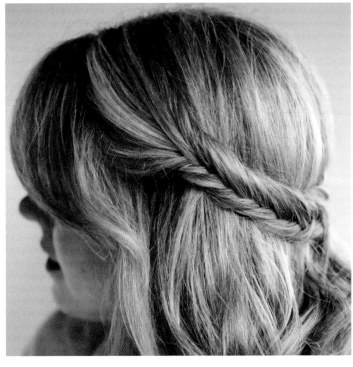

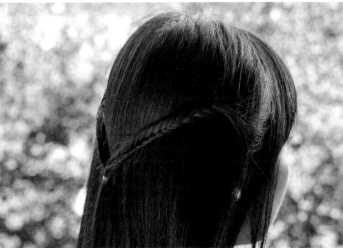

Top: Hairstyling, photography, and modeling by Christina Butcher.
Bottom: Hairstyling and photography by Christina Butcher, modeling by Carolyn Mach.

HOW TO GET IT

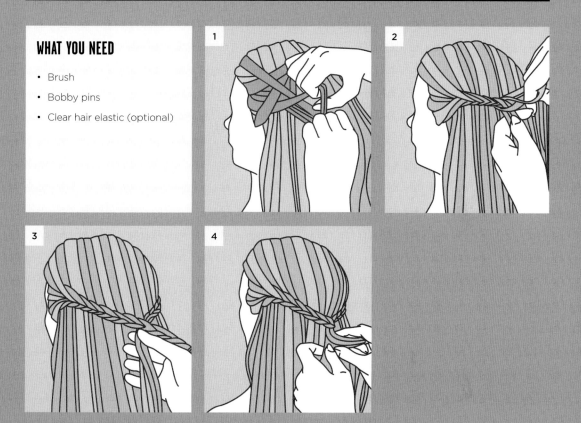

WHAT YOU NEED

- Brush
- Bobby pins
- Clear hair elastic (optional)

1. Start by taking a 1- to 2-inch section of hair near your temple.

2. Split the section in two and start to fishtail braid (see pages 50–51). Keeping one half in each hand, cross a small piece of hair from one section to the other. Keep crossing over small pieces of hair to form the fishtail braid. Once you have braided to the middle of your head, weave a bobby pin through the fishtail and pin to the hair underneath.

3. Repeat the fishtail braid on the opposite side.

4. To join the braids, twist the end of the right braid over and behind the left. Tuck the ends of the hair down and pin in place. Arrange the hair around the crown to disguise the ends of the braids.

TOP TIP

If your hair is fine or very thick and you are having trouble pinning the braids, you can tie them together with a clear hair elastic. Take a small piece of hair from underneath to wrap around the elastic to cover it, then hide the ends of the braids under the rest of your hair to finish off the style.

SIDE FRENCH BRAID
THE LOOK

This loose side version of the French braid will soon become a favorite, and the combination of casual and chic makes it perfect for all sorts of occasions. The side French braid falls diagonally across the back of your head. You'll start the braid at your temple and finish at the nape of your neck on the opposite side. This sweeping braid can finish in either a bun or side ponytail and can be customized according to the length and thickness of your hair.

DIFFICULTY LEVEL
Medium

IDEAL HAIR LENGTH
Medium to long

HAIR EXTENSIONS NEEDED?
No

ASSISTANCE NEEDED?
Yes, but you can do this in your own hair with practice.

ACCESSORIES
You can finish the braid with a pretty bow or add an accessory such as a jeweled pin.

TRY THIS
Experiment with different types of braiding. You could try this style with a detailed small French braid or a French fishtail braid. Customize the end of the braid to suit your hair—if your hair is very long and you can't roll and tuck it underneath, finish in a side bun or side ponytail.

SEE ALSO
French fishtail braid, pages 92–93
Waterfall bun, pages 146–147

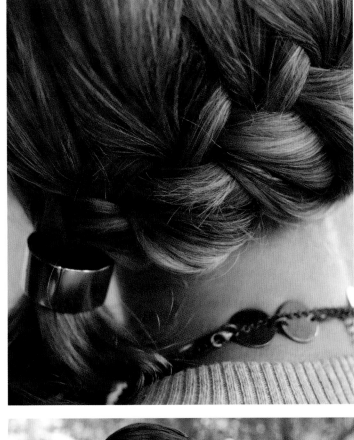

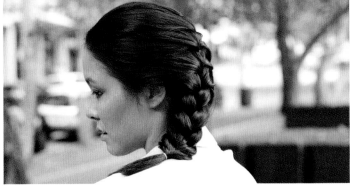

Top: Hairstyling, photography, and modeling by Christina Butcher.
Bottom: Hairstyling by Christina Butcher, photography by Xiaohan Shen, modeling by Tash Williams.

HOW TO GET IT

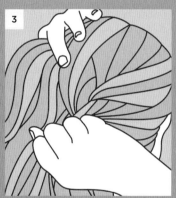

WHAT YOU NEED

- Flat iron
- Brush
- Hair elastic
- Bobby pins

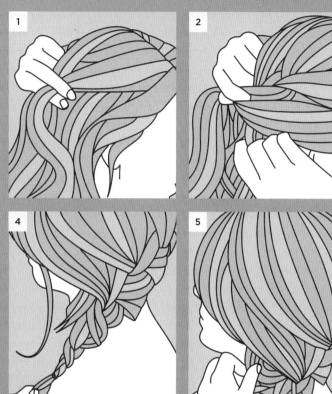

1. It's best to start with straight hair for this hairstyle, so begin by straightening your hair with a flat iron. Brush all of your hair back and make a side part on the right. If you're left-handed, make a side part on the left and braid diagonally to finish at the right side of your neck.

2. Take a section of hair at the right side of your part and split into three equal sections. Begin to French braid (see pages 42–43) diagonally toward the left, adding in very large sections of hair as you go.

3. Keep braiding diagonally until you reach the left side of your head and have no more hair to add.

4. Finish in a basic braid and secure the end with an elastic.

5. Roll up the end of the braid and pin in place underneath your ear.

TOP TIP

This style can work in curly hair, but you'll get a smoother finish in straight hair. Keep the sections of the braid neat, but don't pull it too tight. This style looks best left a little loose.

UNEVEN BRAID
THE LOOK

This simple braiding trick turns what is essentially a regular braid into a completely different style. Uneven braids use the same technique as a basic braid, but instead of weaving three equal sections, you make one section much smaller. It's a cool, slightly unexpected look.

DIFFICULTY LEVEL
Easy

IDEAL HAIR LENGTH
Medium to long

HAIR EXTENSIONS NEEDED?
No

ASSISTANCE NEEDED?
No

ACCESSORIES
Because the final result of this braid is so interesting, there's no need to add more to it, but you could finish the braid with flowers.

TRY THIS
You can use the uneven braiding technique wherever you can do a basic braid. This braid adds a unique twist to low pigtail braids (pages 68–69) or the half-up heart braid (pages 96–97), or you could even roll it up into a bun. For another interesting twist, why not create an uneven braid and use it as one of the sections in a basic braid.

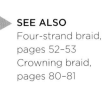
SEE ALSO
Four-strand braid, pages 52–53
Crowning braid, pages 80–81

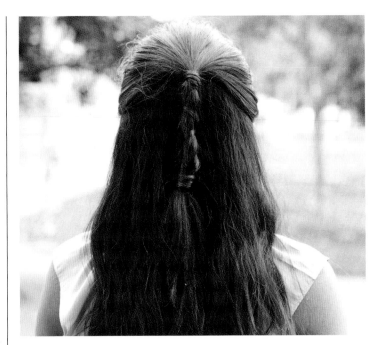

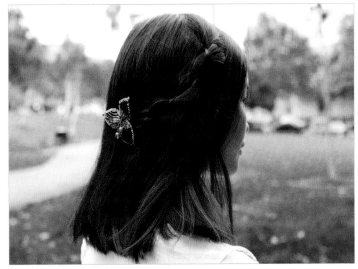

Top: Hairstyling by Christina Butcher, photography by Xiaohan Shen, modeling by Sophia Phan.
Bottom: Hairstyling by Christina Butcher, photography by Xiaohan Shen, modeling by Jessica Tran.

HOW TO GET IT

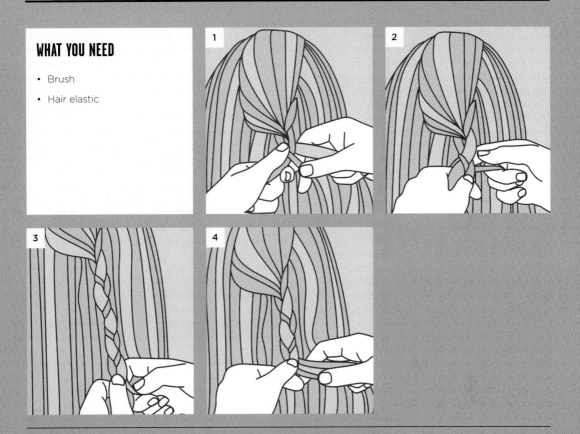

WHAT YOU NEED

- Brush
- Hair elastic

1. Brush your hair to remove any knots and choose a section of hair to work from.

2. Split the section of hair into three: take one very small piece and split the rest into two equal sections.

3. Weave into a basic braid, bringing the right section over the middle, and the left section over the right (now middle).

4. Continue braiding and secure the end with an elastic.

TOP TIP

You can stretch out the two larger sections of the braid to further emphasize the uneven shape. You may find the braid twists as you are weaving it, but this is part of the braid's unique shape, so embrace it! This style is meant to look relaxed, so don't keep the braid too tight-looking. Effortless is best!

FRENCH FISHTAIL BRAID
THE LOOK

This braid is a head-turner. By combining French braiding techniques with the fishtail braid style, you'll create a stunning herringbone-shaped braid. Once you've mastered the regular fishtail braid, you'll love adding the dynamic herringbone shape to your look. Best suited to long hair or hair without layers, this distinctive braid can be worn straight or curved into a gorgeous chignon.

DIFFICULTY LEVEL
Hard

IDEAL HAIR LENGTH
Long

HAIR EXTENSIONS NEEDED?
No

ASSISTANCE NEEDED?
Yes

ACCESSORIES
With so much beautiful detail, this hairstyle doesn't need many accessories, but you can wear a headband to add a pretty touch to the front.

TRY THIS
By braiding your hair on a diagonal angle, you can create a beautiful side French fishtail braid. Curve your braid around to form a fishtail chignon.

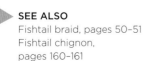

SEE ALSO
Fishtail braid, pages 50–51
Fishtail chignon, pages 160–161

Top: Hairstyling by Christina Butcher, photography by Xiaohan Shen, modeling by Deauvanné.
Bottom left: Hairstyling and makeup by Erin Skipley, photography by Jasmine Star, modeling by Amber Anderson.
Bottom right: Hairstyling and photography by Christina Butcher, modeling by Carolyn Mach.

HOW TO GET IT

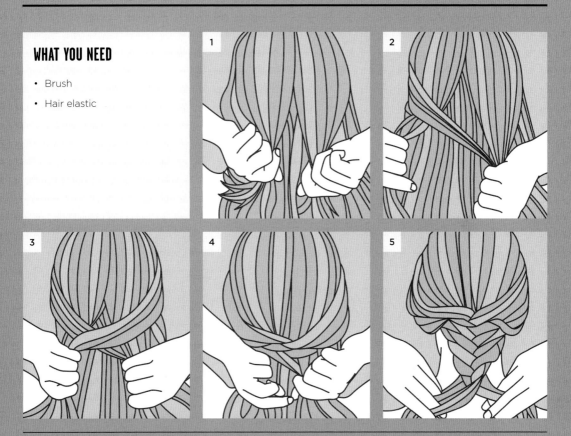

WHAT YOU NEED

- Brush
- Hair elastic

1. Brush your hair to remove any knots. Take a section of hair at the back of your head and split it into two equal sections.

2. Holding one section in each hand, use your index finger to add in hair from the left side of your head and cross it over and add to the right section.

3. Repeat on the right side, picking up hair and adding it to the left section.

4. Continue adding in hair and crossing to the opposite section until there's no more hair left to add.

5. Finish in a regular fishtail braid and secure the end with an elastic.

TOP TIP

This style works best in long hair without too many layers. Try to keep each section small and even to emphasize the herringbone shape. You can also gently pull at the sides of the braid to give it more volume.

ROPE TWIST
THE LOOK

You've heard of a drink with a twist or a story with a twist—well, this is a style with the sweetest twist of all! The rope twist is a classic braid that can be worn on its own or used to add volume to buns and chignons. This simple two-strand braid holds itself together and gives the impression of being a much more complicated style.

DIFFICULTY LEVEL
Medium

IDEAL HAIR LENGTH
Long

HAIR EXTENSIONS NEEDED?
No, but you can use a ponytail extension in short hair.

ASSISTANCE NEEDED?
No

ACCESSORIES
Incorporate a ribbon or scarf into the twist to add some colorful detail: tie around the top of your ponytail and twist the ribbon or scarf in with your rope braid.

TRY THIS
Combine the rope twist with a side ponytail for a pretty variation or turn your rope twist into a top knot or low bun.

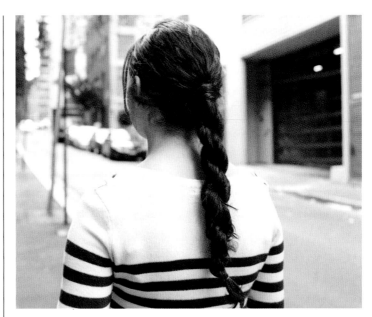

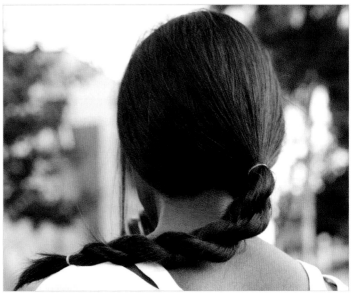

▶ **SEE ALSO**
Coiled bun, pages 148–149
Rope bun, pages 164–165

Top: Hairstyling by Christina Butcher, photography by Xiaohan Shen, modeling by Monica Bowerman .
Bottom: Hairstyling by Christina Butcher, photography by Xiaohan Shen, modeling by Deauvanné .

HOW TO GET IT

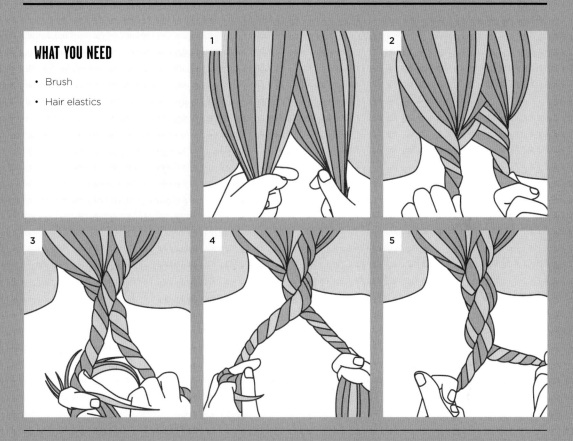

WHAT YOU NEED

- Brush
- Hair elastics

1. Brush your hair to remove any knots and split into two equal sections.

2. Twist each section to the right.

3. Cross the right section of hair over the left section to begin forming the rope twist.

4. Keep twisting the sections to the right and wrapping them to the left.

5. Secure the end of your braid with an elastic.

TOP TIP

Keep twisting the sections to the right so that they keep their shape as you wrap them together. You'll know if you have gone in the wrong direction if the braid falls flat. You can gently stretch out the sides of the braid to make your hair appear thicker.

HALF-UP HEART BRAID
THE LOOK

Wear your heart in your hair with this romantic braid, a clear favorite for a special anniversary or a Valentine's Day dinner. Braiding shapes into your hair can be great fun, and they add an extra dimension to ordinary braided styles. After you've mastered this heart shape, why not try some shape ideas of your own?

DIFFICULTY LEVEL
Medium

IDEAL HAIR LENGTH
Medium to long

HAIR EXTENSIONS NEEDED?
No

ASSISTANCE NEEDED?
Yes, but you can do this in your own hair with practice.

ACCESSORIES
Your hair forms the focus in this hairstyle, so no adornments are needed.

TRY THIS
You can create a heart in your hair wherever you can make two braids, such as at the side of your head. This hairstyle also looks great when you braid two hearts next to each other.

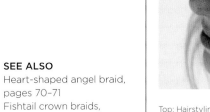

SEE ALSO
Heart-shaped angel braid, pages 70–71
Fishtail crown braids, pages 86–87

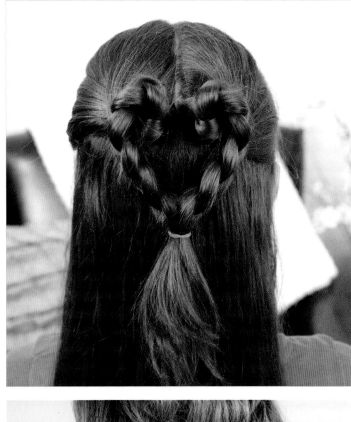

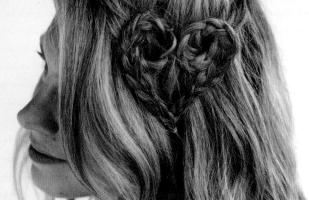

Top: Hairstyling, photography, and modeling by Mindy McKnight.
Bottom: Hairstyling, photography, and modeling by Christina Butcher.

HOW TO GET IT

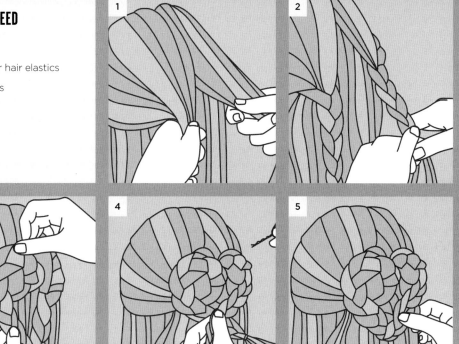

WHAT YOU NEED

- Brush
- Small clear hair elastics
- Bobby pins

1. Brush your hair and section off the top half of your hair. Split into two equal sections.

2. Braid each section using the basic braid technique and secure the ends with small clear elastics.

3. Loop the left-hand braid up and around to form the top of the heart. Pin in place with bobby pins.

4. Repeat with the right-hand braid, coiling it around to form the top of the heart. Use bobby pins to secure it in place.

5. You can finish either in a ponytail by removing the elastics from the ends of each braid and securing them together with one elastic, or by folding the tails of each braid up to form the point of the heart. Tuck in any loose ends and pin in place with bobby pins.

TOP TIP

Use clear elastics or elastics that match your hair color, as they will be less conspicuous in the heart shape. If you have very long hair, the braids can be folded in half before forming the heart.

SCARF BRAID
THE LOOK

A scarf braid is a simple way to add color to your hairstyle while making your hair look thicker at the same time. This chic, carefree summer style offers you a new way to wear your favorite scarf and is a great choice for alfresco dining or a day out on the water.

DIFFICULTY LEVEL
Easy

IDEAL HAIR LENGTH
Long

HAIR EXTENSIONS NEEDED?
No, but you can use a ponytail extension if required.

ASSISTANCE NEEDED?
No

ACCESSORIES
You can use any scarf to add color and style to a plain braid, but light silk scarves are best, and choose a length that is close to your hair length.

TRY THIS
If you have a longer scarf, you can tie it around your head as a headband first before adding it to your braid. You can also add a scarf into any braid to make your hair look thicker. Try it in a braided bun, a crown braid, or Heidi braids.

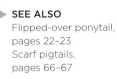
SEE ALSO
Flipped-over ponytail, pages 22–23
Scarf pigtails, pages 66–67

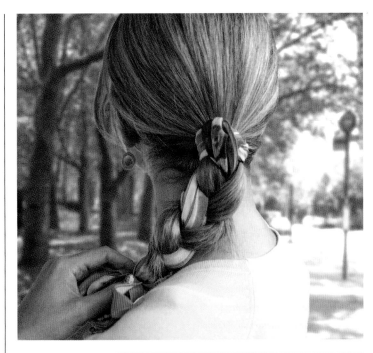

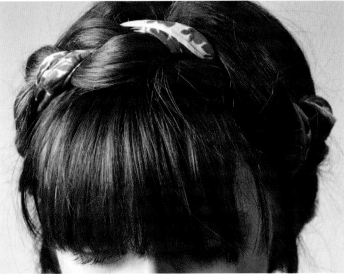

Top: Hairstyling, photography, and modeling by Christina Butcher.
Bottom: Hairstyling, photography, and modeling by Bailey Tan.

HOW TO GET IT

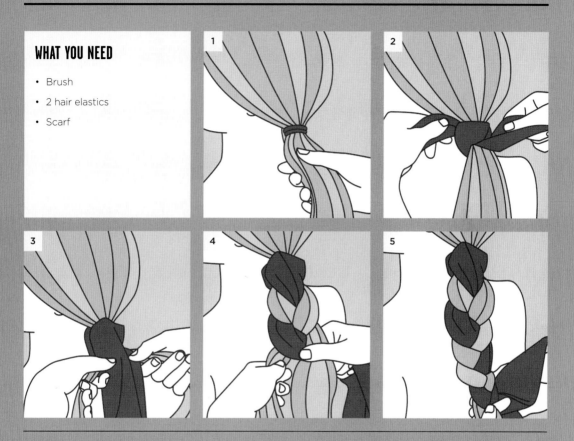

WHAT YOU NEED

- Brush
- 2 hair elastics
- Scarf

1. Brush your hair back into a ponytail and secure with an elastic.

2. Tie your scarf around the base of your ponytail.

3. Split your ponytail into two equal sections and use the scarf as the third section in your braid.

4. Cross the left over the middle, and the right over the left (now middle), and continue braiding all the way down.

5. Secure the end of your hair (and the scarf) with an elastic.

TOP TIP

If using a square scarf, fold it in half to form a triangle, and then continue folding it over to create a long ribbon. Tie it to the base of your ponytail with the loose end underneath so it won't show. Make the scarf the center section of the braid. If your scarf is too long, you can tie it into a bow at the end of your braid.

SLIDE-UP BRAID
THE LOOK

This braid looks complicated, but if you can do a basic braid, you'll be able to master the slide-up braid with ease. For this style you'll hold one piece of the braid and slide the other two sections. The slide-up braid is also known as a snake braid because it gives the effect of the braid weaving its way along a single section of hair—just like a snake weaves around a branch! This elaborate-looking braid is good for any occasion, formal or informal, work or play.

DIFFICULTY LEVEL
Easy

IDEAL HAIR LENGTH
Medium to long

HAIR EXTENSIONS NEEDED?
No

ASSISTANCE NEEDED?
No

ACCESSORIES
Add your favorite clips or barrettes for a beautiful finish.

TRY THIS
Use the slide-up technique in any hairstyle where you can do a basic braid, such as a side braid (see pages 84–85) or crowning braid (see pages 80–81).

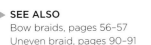
SEE ALSO
Bow braids, pages 56–57
Uneven braid, pages 90–91

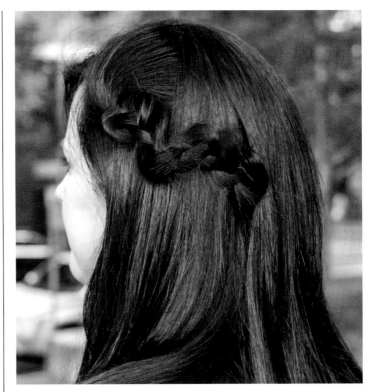

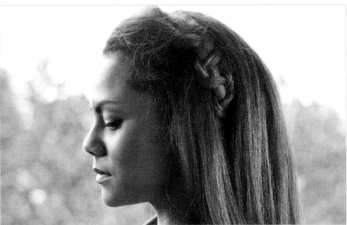

Top: Hairstyling and photography by Christina Butcher, modeling by Ashleigh Forster.
Bottom: Hairstyling by Christina Butcher, photography by Xiaohan Shen, modeling by Dorothy Jean Joly.

HOW TO GET IT

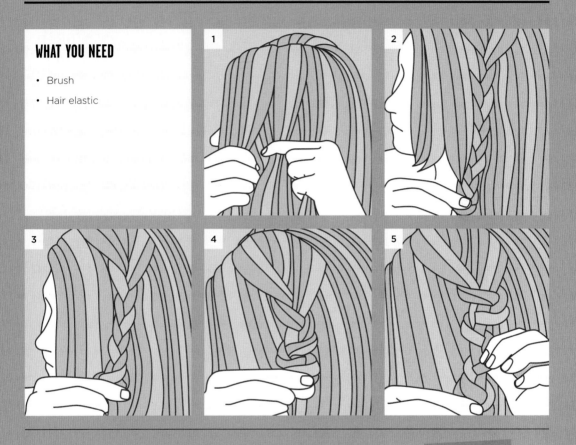

WHAT YOU NEED

- Brush
- Hair elastic

1. Brush your hair and section off a piece for your braid.

2. Split the section into three equal pieces and do a basic braid all the way down to the end.

3. Take the end of your braid and hold one piece (it doesn't matter which one) with one hand and slide the other two sections up with your other hand.

4. The braid will gather and bunch initially, but pull each turn of the braid up along the central section to even it out.

5. Adjust the braid all the way up to sit evenly, and secure the end with a clear elastic.

TOP TIP

Don't be scared to slide the braid right up, as you can always adjust it back down and make it more evenly spaced. Don't braid too tightly, as this will make it harder to slide the braid up.

WATERFALL BRAID
THE LOOK

This style uses the French braiding technique, but instead of picking up a new section of hair from the bottom, you allow it to flow through, creating a cascading waterfall effect. This braid can be done in any length of hair, from chin-length bob to very long. The stunning waterfall braid is perfect for long days on the beach and casual outdoor parties and is a gorgeous choice for the boho bride. It takes some practice to perfect but looks fabulous when you get it right!

DIFFICULTY LEVEL
Hard

IDEAL HAIR LENGTH
Any

HAIR EXTENSIONS NEEDED?
No

ASSISTANCE NEEDED?
Yes, but you can do this in your own hair with practice.

ACCESSORIES
The beauty of this braid lies in the elegant falling sections, so you don't have to decorate this style further. For a sweet touch you could finish the braid off with a simple ribbon or weave a daisy chain through the waterfall.

TRY THIS
You can start from the left and work right, depending on which side you prefer to part your hair. This braid forms part of the waterfall bun and can be doubled up to form a double waterfall braid.

▶ **SEE ALSO**
Angel braid, pages 48–49
Waterfall bun, pages 146–147

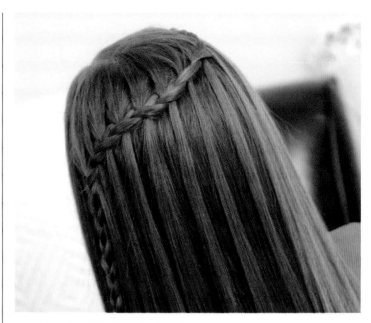

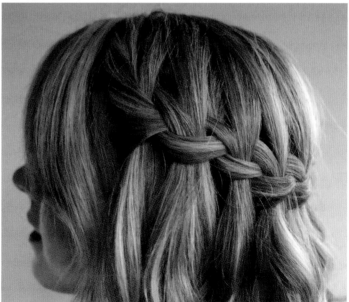

Top: Hairstyling, photography, and modeling by Mindy McKnight.
Bottom: Hairstyling, photography, and modeling by Christina Butcher.

HOW TO GET IT

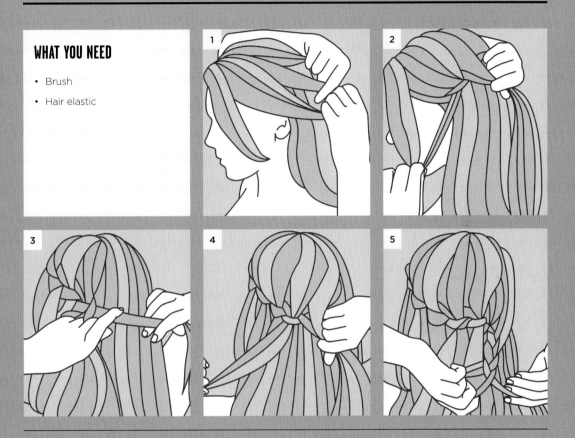

WHAT YOU NEED

- Brush
- Hair elastic

1. Brush all of your hair back and away from your face. If you have bangs, you can leave them out. To start, take a 1- to 2-inch section of hair from the left side of your head and split it into three equal parts.

2. Begin braiding by crossing section 1 over 2 and then section 3 over 1. Add in hair from the top of your head to section 2 and then cross it over section 3.

3. Next, instead of crossing section 1 over 2, drop it out and pick up a new piece of hair from just behind it. Cross this over section 2 and continue braiding.

4. Only add in hair from the top, and drop out the bottom piece as you go, remembering to pick up a new piece from behind it.

5. When you reach the right side, stop adding in hair, finish off the waterfall braid, and secure with an elastic (see the Top Tip for finishing ideas).

TOP TIP

There are two ways to finish off your waterfall braid: in a regular braid or in a loose ponytail. Reach your arm right over your head when you start, and every time you grab a section of hair from the top of your head, add it to the braid, let it drop, and replace it with a new section.

DOUBLE WATERFALL BRAID
THE LOOK

This hairstyle creates a double layer of waterfall braids by incorporating the "falling" parts of the braid twice. You'll do this by making two separate braids, one above the other, or by making a single braid that turns and repeats under the first braid in a sweeping fashion. Because of its complexity and intricacy, this style would be a great look for a special event like a wedding or a significant birthday—in other words, a time when you'll be photographed a lot!

DIFFICULTY LEVEL
Hard

IDEAL HAIR LENGTH
Medium to long

HAIR EXTENSIONS NEEDED?
No

ASSISTANCE NEEDED?
Yes, but you can do this in your own hair with practice.

ACCESSORIES
This elegant braid doesn't need any further decoration, but you can finish the waterfall braids in regular braids and add small bows at the end of each.

TRY THIS
You can either create this look with two separate braids, one above the other, or by turning your waterfall braid around and incorporating the falling parts in the braid below. Instead of letting the top section fall through the second braid, combine it into a Dutch braid for a faux bob finish.

▶ **SEE ALSO**
Mermaid braid, pages 62–63
Waterfall twist braid, pages 110–111

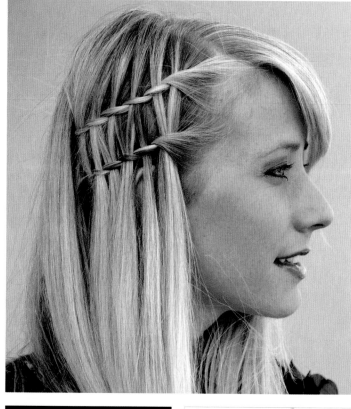

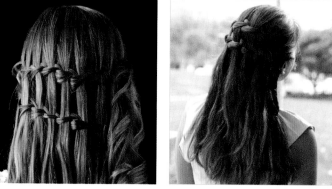

Top: Hairstyling, photography, and modeling by Abby Smith/Twist Me Pretty.
Bottom left: Hairstyling and photography by Erica Gray Beauty Company, modeling by Joanna Wilkinson.
Bottom right: Hairstyling and photography by Christina Butcher, modeling by Sophia Phan.

HOW TO GET IT

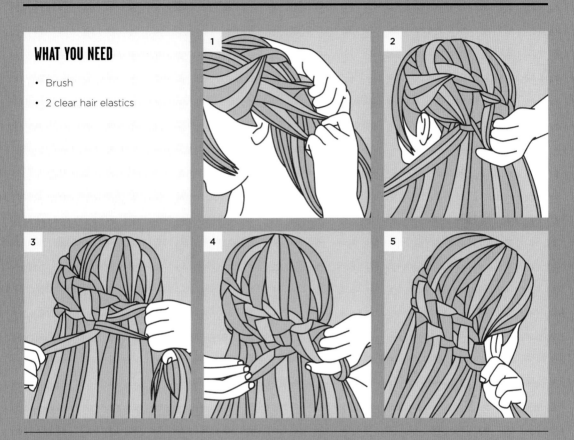

WHAT YOU NEED

- Brush
- 2 clear hair elastics

1. Brush your hair and make a waterfall braid across the back of your head (see pages 102–103). Use a clear elastic to secure the ends of the braid and leave the rest in a loose ponytail.

2. Start the second waterfall braid 1 to 2 inches below the start of the first braid. Take a 1- to 2-inch section of hair and split it into three.

3. Braid together, crossing section 1 over 2, then section 3 over 1. Add the first cascading section from the first waterfall braid into section 2 and cross it over section 3.

4. Instead of using section 1 to cross over 2, drop it out, and pick up a new piece of hair from behind it. Cross this over section 2 and continue the braid. Continue, adding in the falling pieces of hair from the top waterfall braid, dropping out the bottom piece, and picking up a new piece just behind it.

5. When you reach the right side, stop adding in hair and secure both braids together with a small clear elastic, or finish in a basic braid.

TOP TIP

The key to this style is to include the falling sections from the top braid into the braid below. When braiding someone else's hair it's much clearer to see which sections to add. To keep track of this in your own hair, you can section off each cascading piece with an elastic.

LACE BRAID
THE LOOK

The lace braid is a half French braid with a delicate scalloped edge. By brushing your hair forward you can create a braided layer of hair that frames your face. The way the long sections come down to meet the braid on your hairline makes this style look like an upside-down waterfall braid.

DIFFICULTY LEVEL
Medium

IDEAL HAIR LENGTH
Medium to long

HAIR EXTENSIONS NEEDED?
No

ASSISTANCE NEEDED?
Yes, but you can do this in your own hair with practice.

ACCESSORIES
You could weave a fine ribbon through the braid to give the style an extra accent of pretty! Finish the braid with a small bow or decorative band.

TRY THIS
This braid looks beautiful if you start with a center part and mirror the braid on both sides around your face.

▶ **SEE ALSO**
Angel braid, pages 48–49
Side braid, pages 84–85

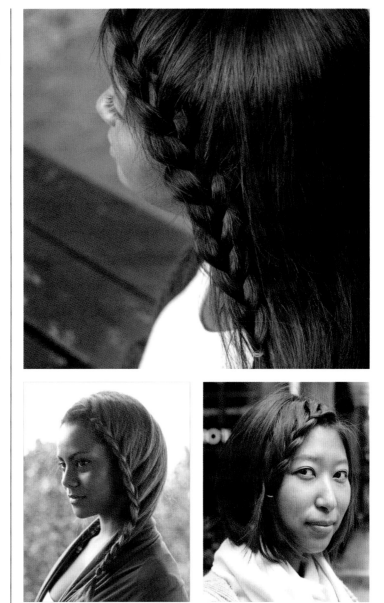

Top: Hairstyling and photography by Christina Butcher, modeling by Nicole Jeyaraj.
Bottom left: Hairstyling and photography by Christina Butcher, modeling by Dorothy Jean Joly.
Bottom right: Hairstyling by Christina Butcher, photography by Xiaohan Shen, modeling by Hitomi Nakajima.

HOW TO GET IT

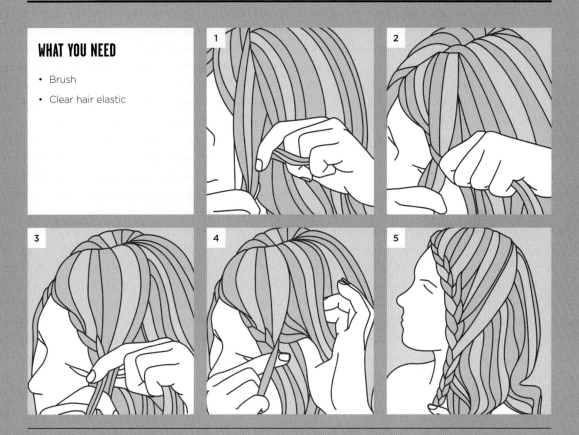

WHAT YOU NEED

- Brush
- Clear hair elastic

1. Brush your hair and make a deep side part on the right side of your head. Take a small section of hair at the start of the part and split it into three.

2. Start the French braid here, but only add in hair from behind (not from your hairline).

3–4. Keep adding in very small sections to your braid until you reach your cheekbone or jaw line.

5. Finish in a regular braid and secure with a clear elastic.

TOP TIP

Angle the braid right onto your face and in front of your hairline. You want the braid to sit grazing the edge of your eyebrow and come down the left side of your face.

DUTCH CROWN BRAIDS
THE LOOK

Dutch crown braids create a crown of hair that sits on and over your hairline, and is one of the prettiest ways to wear your hair up. This style is great if you don't like to show your ears, as you can pull the braids forward to sit over the top of them. Dutch crown braids are formed by making a diagonal part down the back of your head, and two Dutch braids, starting at the part, circle around your head and follow your hairline. Finishing in pigtails at the back, the ends curve round to complete the crown. This style perfectly frames the face, making it a gorgeous look for any occasion.

DIFFICULTY LEVEL
Hard

IDEAL HAIR LENGTH
Medium to long

HAIR EXTENSIONS NEEDED?
No

ASSISTANCE NEEDED?
Yes, but you can do this in your own hair with practice.

ACCESSORIES
For an extra-romantic look, sit a flower crown behind your Dutch crown braids. You can weave fresh flowers through your braid or add small diamanté pins for a little sparkle.

TRY THIS
This type of crown braid is perfect for very long hair, as you can pin the braid all the way round to create a double crown.

 SEE ALSO
Grecian braid, pages 78–79
Upside-down braid bun, pages 136–137

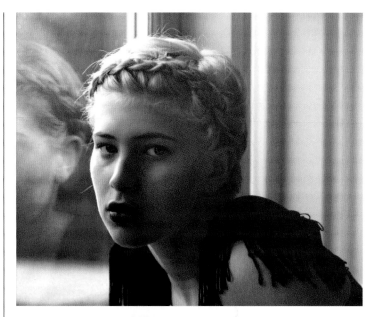

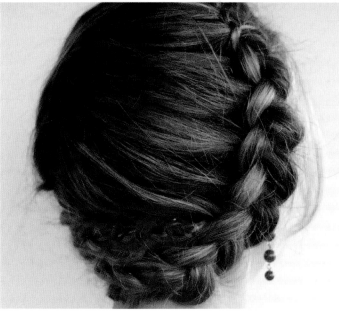

Top: Hairstyling, photography, and modeling by Suzy Wimbourne Photography.
Bottom: Hairstyling, photography, and modeling by Christina Butcher.

HOW TO GET IT

WHAT YOU NEED

- Brush
- Tail comb
- Hair clip
- 2 clear hair elastics
- Bobby pins
- Hairpins (optional)

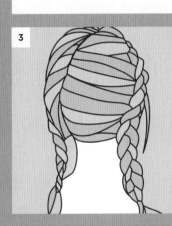

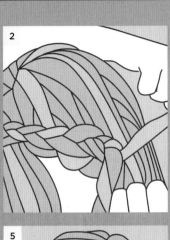

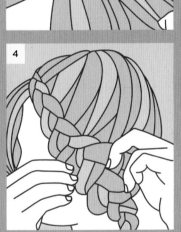

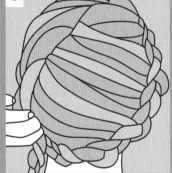

1. Brush your hair and with your tail comb, make a deep side part on the right side of your head, and run the part diagonally across the back of your head to the left side of your neck. Clip away the right section of hair so that it's out of the way.

2. Take a 1-inch section of hair on the left side of the part and split into three. If you have bangs, you can leave them out or add them in. Start to form a Dutch braid (see pages 44–45) following your hairline, but only add in sections from along the part line, not from your hairline.

3. Keep the Dutch braid going all the way round your hairline, adding in hair from the part line. When you reach your neck, finish in a regular braid and secure with a clear elastic. Repeat the Dutch braid on the other side of your part, braiding all the way around your hairline and finishing in a regular braid.

4. To finish the style, stretch the braids out.

5. Pin each braid up into the opposite braid and tuck the ends underneath.

TOP TIP

Angle the braid as close as possible to your hairline. As you braid, keep your hair taut and ensure the braid frames your face. You can then further stretch your braids to sit out and over your ears (if you want to cover them up!).

WATERFALL TWIST BRAID
THE LOOK

The waterfall twist is a variation of the waterfall braid. Instead of braiding with three sections, however, you braid with just two, and the falling waterfall sections drop between the twists without being incorporated into the actual braid. Because this is a more informal version of the waterfall braid, it's perfect for more relaxed situations—an evening with friends, a day with family—but it will receive just the same amount of attention.

DIFFICULTY LEVEL
Medium

IDEAL HAIR LENGTH
Medium to long

HAIR EXTENSIONS NEEDED?
No

ASSISTANCE NEEDED?
Yes, but you can do this in your own hair with practice.

ACCESSORIES
Clip a bow or pretty barrette to the end of the waterfall twist. Ribbon can also be weaved through the finished braid to add color and draw attention to the twist.

TRY THIS
If your hair is long, try stretching one twist all the way around your head.

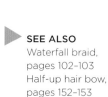

SEE ALSO
Waterfall braid, pages 102–103
Half-up hair bow, pages 152–153

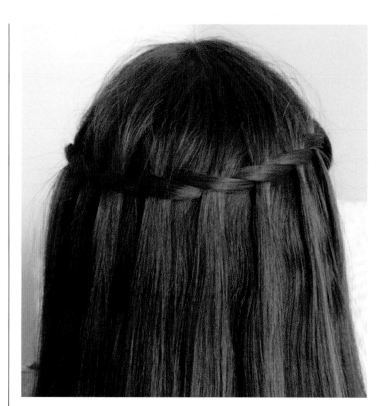

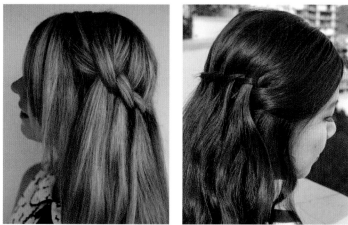

Top: Hairstyling, photography, and modeling by Mindy McKnight.
Bottom left: Hairstyling, photography, and modeling by Christina Butcher.
Bottom right: Hairstyling and photography by Christina Butcher, modeling by An Ly.

HOW TO GET IT

WHAT YOU NEED

- Brush
- Hair elastic
- Bobby pins

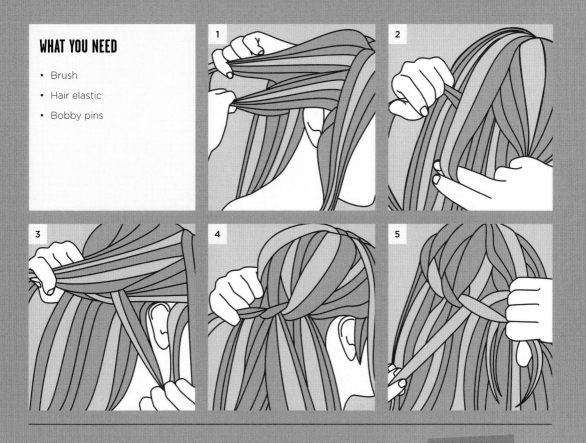

1. Start by brushing all of your hair through to remove any knots and catches, and then take a large section on the right side of your head. Split this into two equal sections and twist the top section around the bottom section.

2. Take a section of hair from above the twist and place it in between the two twisting pieces. It doesn't connect, it just goes straight through.

3. Twist the two original pieces. Take another section from above the twist and place it in between again. Keep twisting and placing new pieces of hair in between each twist. You should get three to four twists.

4. When you reach the back center of your head, twist the two sections around again and weave a bobby pin through to secure the braid to the back of your head.

5. Repeat on the other side, twisting and adding sections that fall through the twists. When you reach the back where the right braid finishes, add one more section through, twist together, and pin in place.

TOP TIP

Be sure the sections that fall through the twists are the same size; if they're different, the braid will look uneven. As you're not really adding any hair into this braid other than the two original sections, make sure you take a large enough section to twist.

PRETZEL BRAID
THE LOOK

This pretty twist on pigtails is a fun way to wear your hair up. Two pigtail braids twist around each other in a pretzel shape that sits low at the back of your head. This style doesn't have to be precise—the idea is to create a nice curved shape from the braid. The look is cool, modern, and distinctive and complements any outfit.

DIFFICULTY LEVEL
Medium

IDEAL HAIR LENGTH
Long

HAIR EXTENSIONS NEEDED?
No

ASSISTANCE NEEDED?
Yes, but you can do this in your own hair with practice.

ACCESSORIES
Because this is a decorative braid, you don't want to overdo it with more accessories. A simple pin at the center of the pretzel draws attention to your braid.

TRY THIS
Once you've mastered this version, try creating other shapes and styles with your pigtails. You can also try the pretzel style using the fishtail braid (see pages 50–51) or uneven braid (see pages 90–91) techniques.

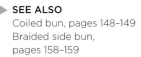

SEE ALSO
Coiled bun, pages 148–149
Braided side bun, pages 158–159

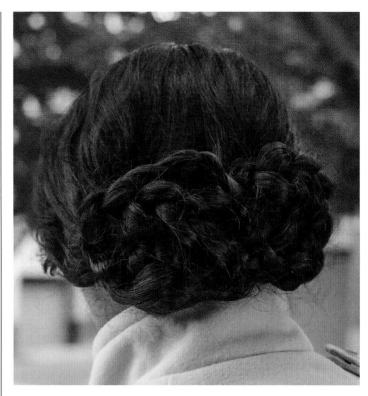

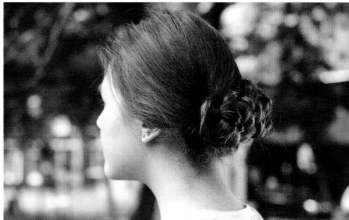

Top: Hairstyling and photography by Christina Butcher, modeling by Tanu Vasu.
Bottom: Hairstyling by Christina Butcher, photography by Xiaohan Shen, modeling by Sophia Phan.

HOW TO GET IT

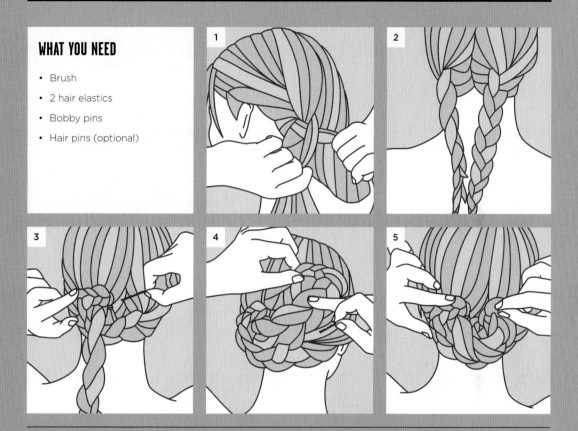

WHAT YOU NEED

- Brush
- 2 hair elastics
- Bobby pins
- Hair pins (optional)

1. Brush your hair and split it down the middle into two equal sections.

2. Braid both sections into pigtails and secure the ends with elastics.

3. Cross one braid over the other. Take the braid that's now below and twist it around the other braid to create a "C" shape. Pin in place with bobby pins.

4. Repeat with the other braid, curving it up and around to make the same shape, and pin in place.

5. Adjust your braids to sit in a kind of pretzel or knot shape at the back of your head. Tuck the ends of your braids behind the knot and pin them using bobby pins. Use hairpins to secure the style if you have thick hair.

TOP TIP

Start your pigtails a little higher on your head so that you have more space to arrange your pretzel-shaped bun. If you need help keeping your braids in place, you can section your hair with elastics before braiding, but remember to remove the top elastics before assembling the pretzel shape.

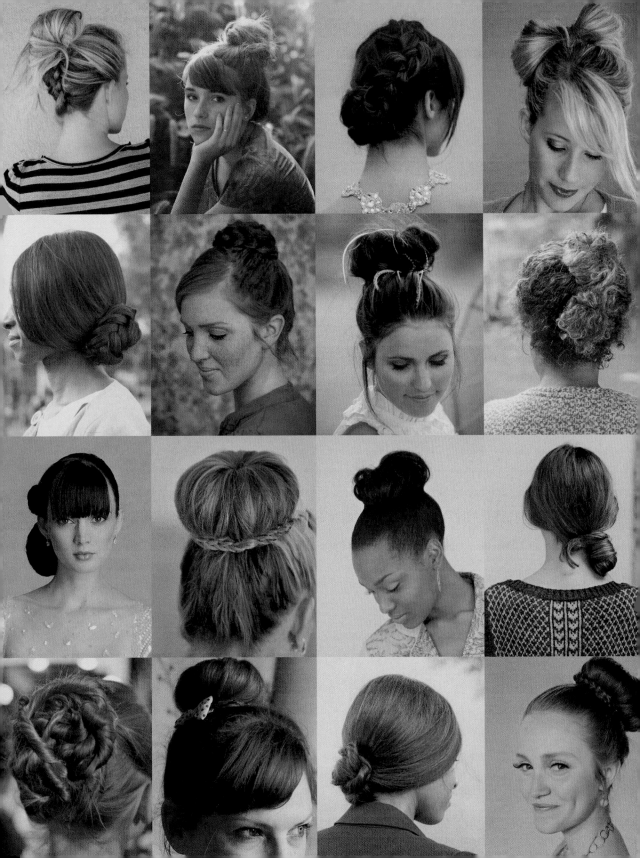

CHAPTER 3
BUNS, KNOTS, AND TWISTS

TOP KNOT BUN
THE LOOK

So French, so chic! The top knot is an effortless hairstyle that always looks stylish. It's quick and easy to do and an ideal way to hide less-than-perfect hair while still maintaining some fashion cred. The cool top knot sits high on the crown of your head, adding great height to your look. The top knot looks and holds best in second-day hair.

DIFFICULTY LEVEL
Easy

IDEAL HAIR LENGTH
Long

HAIR EXTENSIONS NEEDED?
No

ASSISTANCE NEEDED?
No

ACCESSORIES
Top knot buns are a fabulous base for all kinds of accessories. Headbands add instant detail to the front, and you can add flowers, scarves, or bows to accessorize the bun at the back.

TRY THIS
Wear it messy for an effortless look, or try one of the variations of the top knot bun in this chapter for extra detail, such as the donut bun or braided bun.

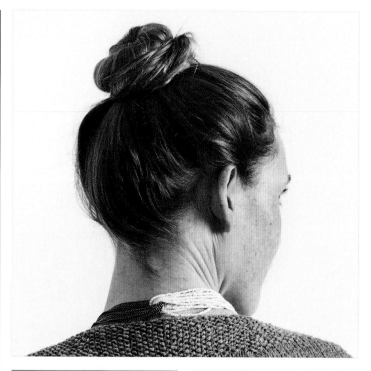

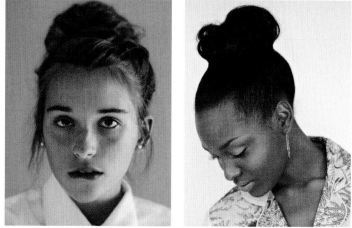

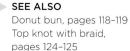 **SEE ALSO**
Donut bun, pages 118–119
Top knot with braid, pages 124–125

Top: Photograph courtesy of Brooklyn Tweed. Hairstyling by Stephanie Gelot and Aine Vonnegut, photography by Jared Flood, modeling by Aine Vonnegut.
Bottom left: Hairstyling, photography, and modeling by Alison Titus.
Bottom right: Photograph courtesy of Plum Pretty Sugar. Hairstyling by Makeup 1011 and Katie M, photography by Marisa Holmes.

HOW TO GET IT

WHAT YOU NEED

- Brush
- Hair elastic
- Bobby pins or hairpins
- Hairspray (optional)

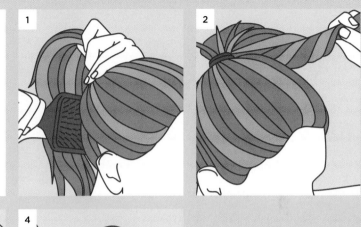

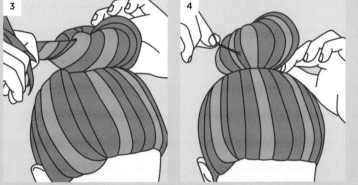

1. Brush your hair and gather it up into a high ponytail. Secure with a strong elastic.

2. Loosely twist your hair and then loop it around the base of the ponytail. If you have long hair, you may need to loop it around twice, but don't pull your hair too tight, because you want the bun to be a little loose.

3. Secure the base of the bun with bobby pins or hairpins.

4. If required, finish with a spritz of hairspray to hold any flyaways and loose pieces of hair.

TOP TIP

You need only four bobby pins to secure the bun—one at both the front and back and one at each side. If your hair is thick, use hairpins to pin the bun in place instead. Don't try to be too precise with top knots—if they're too tight, they can give you a headache, and remember, you still want to look effortless.

DONUT BUN
THE LOOK

This bun has a little secret . . . padding! Donut-shaped mesh padding adds a little oomph and turns your top knot into a statement—think of it like a push up bra for your hair. This style is also known as a sock bun. It takes its name from a DIY trick where you make your own padding with an old sock. Simply cut the toe section off the end of a sock so you are left with a tube. Roll the tube up into a donut shape and you have the perfect fit for your bun! You can also purchase hair padding in lots of shapes, sizes, and colors from beauty retailers. With this hidden secret, everyone will think you have thick, long hair, so it's a great look for those with fine or short hair.

DIFFICULTY LEVEL
Medium

IDEAL HAIR LENGTH
Medium to long

HAIR EXTENSIONS NEEDED?
No

ASSISTANCE NEEDED?
No

ACCESSORIES
Like the top knot bun, the donut bun loves an accessory. Tie scarves around the bun or add clips, barrettes, flowers, or headbands.

TRY THIS
Try a low donut bun at the nape of your neck, or wear it to the side for an asymmetrical look.

▶ **SEE ALSO**
Pillow bun, pages 154–155
Braided side bun, pages 158–159

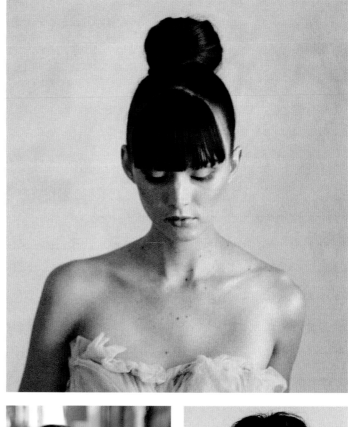

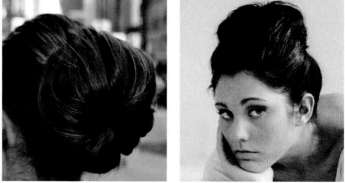

Top: Hairstyling and makeup by Erin Skipley, photography by Elizabeth Messina, modeling by Faye.
Bottom left: Hairstyling and modeling by Chrissann Gasparro, photography by Drew Nebrig.
Bottom right: Hairstyling by Flavia Carolina with Versa Artistry, photography by Yan Photo.

HOW TO GET IT

WHAT YOU NEED

- Paddle brush or bristle brush
- Hair elastic
- Hair donut
- Comb
- Bobby pins
- Hairspray

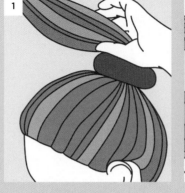

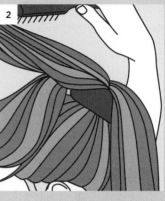

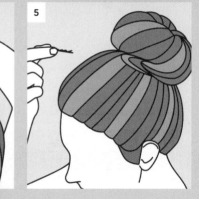

1. Using a paddle or bristle brush, gather all your hair up into a high ponytail and secure it with a strong elastic. You'll need your ponytail to stay secure and support your bun. Pop your donut padding around your ponytail. Try and use padding that is close in color to your hair color.

2. Gently backcomb your ponytail to create more volume so you have enough hair to cover the donut.

3. Hide the donut by twisting and wrapping your hair around it.

4. Find the center of your ponytail and wrap your hair around evenly to cover the donut. Use bobby pins to secure the ends of your hair. You can also tuck your hair under the donut to keep it neat.

5. Finish with a spritz of hairspray to smooth any frizzy flyaways.

TOP TIP

Keep your donut bun a little messy and natural looking, and no one will know you are hiding secret padding in there. Tease the ponytail first to add texture to the finished style and pull at a few sections of hair to keep it looking a little uneven. If you want to use a real sock, remember to wash it first. Pooh!

FISHTAIL BRAIDED BUN
THE LOOK

Amp up the texture in your top knot with this fishtail braided bun. This hairstyle works best in long hair, but you can use extensions or padding to add more volume to the finished look. The braid is made up of two fishtail braids that twist around to form a top knot. You can't really tell that it's a fishtail braid when it's finished, but you can see the beautiful herringbone texture of the braid. Fishtail braids are traditionally messy, so be prepared for the bun to be messy too. This is an excellent look for a fun day out with friends.

DIFFICULTY LEVEL
Medium

IDEAL HAIR LENGTH
Long

HAIR EXTENSIONS NEEDED?
No

ASSISTANCE NEEDED?
Yes

ACCESSORIES
With so much detail in the fishtail braided bun, you can keep it simple with your hair accessories. A classic barrette or headband is all that's needed to dress up this hairstyle.

TRY THIS
If you have very long hair, you can just do one braid and wind it all the way around to form the bun. Alternatively, try braiding three or four smaller fishtail braids and twist them up into a more detailed bun.

SEE ALSO
Fishtail braid, pages 50–51
Braided top bun, pages 170–171

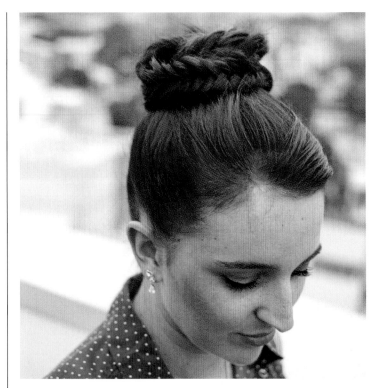

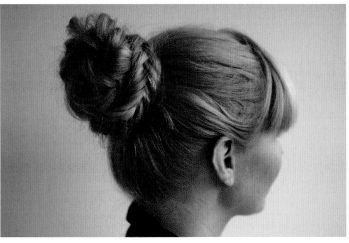

Top: Hairstyling and photography by Christina Butcher, modeling by Elly Hanson.
Bottom: Hairstyling and photography by Christina Butcher, modeling by Michaela Williams.

HOW TO GET IT

WHAT YOU NEED

- Paddle brush or bristle brush
- Strong hair elastic
- Hair clip
- 2 small clear hair elastics
- Bobby pins

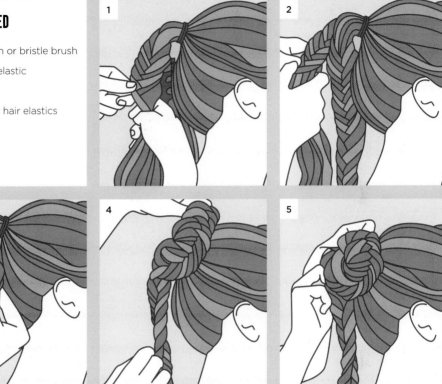

1. Brush your hair using a paddle or bristle brush and gather it into a high ponytail. Secure with a strong hair elastic.

2. Split your ponytail in two and clip away one half. Split the other section in two and begin to fishtail braid (see pages 50–51). Secure the end of the braid with a small clear elastic. Repeat, fishtail braiding the other half of your ponytail.

3. Stretch out your fishtail braids.

4. Take the first braid and twist it up and around the base of your ponytail and pin in place with bobby pins.

5. Repeat step 4 with the second braid, twisting in the opposite direction to create a full bun. Secure the bun with bobby pins.

TOP TIP

Stretching out your braids before twisting them into the bun emphasizes the delicate shape of the braids and adds more detail to the finished bun. You can still adjust the bun once it is pinned in place, but it's easier to shape the braids beforehand.

MESSY HIGH BUN
THE LOOK

Look like you had the best night of your life and just woke up in Paris with the messy high bun. In fact, the lazier you are, the easier this style is—the dirtier your hair, the better the messy high bun will look! If your hair is squeaky clean, use a texturizing powder or sea salt spray to mess it up before starting this hairstyle. It's a look that embraces flyaways, so bear that in mind with whatever your plans are. This is a great casual hairstyle, but not necessarily ideal for more formal or work occasions.

DIFFICULTY LEVEL
Easy

IDEAL HAIR LENGTH
Long

HAIR EXTENSIONS NEEDED?
No

ASSISTANCE NEEDED?
No

ACCESSORIES
This hairstyle looks effortless because it is! There's therefore no need to go over the top with accessories. A headband or thin ribbon can help to adorn this bun, but keep it simple and chic.

TRY THIS
The messy high bun is even easier to do if you have naturally curly or wavy hair, and is perfect in second-day hair. The messy bun can also be worn low on the nape of the neck, or to the side.

SEE ALSO
Side ponytail, pages 18–19
Messy ponytail, pages 32–33

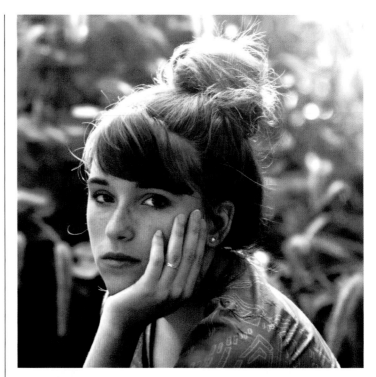

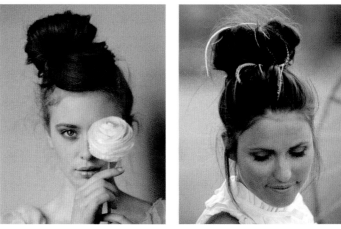

Top: Hairstyling, photography, and modeling by Alison Titus.
Bottom left: Hairstyling and makeup by Erin Skipley, photography by Elizabeth Messina, modeling by Ashlyn Pearce.
Bottom right: Photograph courtesy of Fine Featherheads. Photography by Kate Broussard, Soulshots Photography.

HOW TO GET IT

WHAT YOU NEED

- Dry shampoo
- Hair donut
- Hair elastic
- Comb
- Bobby pins
- Hairpins (optional)

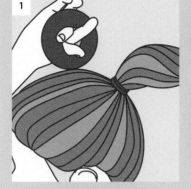

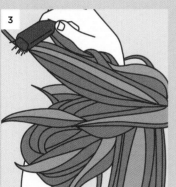

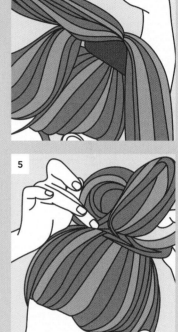

1. Spray dry shampoo onto your hair to give it some texture and body. You want the finished style to look loose and relaxed, so don't brush your hair. Use your fingertips to gather all your hair up into a high ponytail and secure with a hair elastic. Place the hair donut at the base of your ponytail.

2-3. Backcomb your ponytail to create even more mess and texture.

4. Gently twist your ponytail and curve it around the base of your ponytail to form a bun. Use bobby pins to secure the bun in place. If your hair is thick or curly, try using hairpins for a stronger hold.

5. Pull some pieces of hair loose around your face and at the nape of your neck to give this style a "lived-in" look.

TOP TIP

Dry shampoo is the perfect styling product for creating this hairstyle, whether your hair is clean or dirty. It absorbs oil at the roots of your hair and adds a matte texture to the midlengths and ends.

TOP KNOT WITH BRAID
THE LOOK

Take your top knot to the next level and let your hair be your accessory in this look. For this style you simply wind a braid around the base of your high bun. Depending on the length and thickness of your hair, you can start with a top knot or donut bun, and leave a section out to braid around the bun base. This technique offers a simple way to dress up a regular, everyday bun.

DIFFICULTY LEVEL
Medium

IDEAL HAIR LENGTH
Long

HAIR EXTENSIONS NEEDED?
No

ASSISTANCE NEEDED?
No

ACCESSORIES
A simple headband or clip adds detail, but the braid is the real accessory in this hairstyle. For an evening look, a beaded or jeweled barrette can be added to the back of the bun. Small jeweled pins can also be added down the center of the braid for some added sparkle.

TRY THIS
Instead of a basic braid around the base of your bun, try a fishtail braid. You can even do two or three very thin braids and wrap them around for added detail. You can also wear this bun to the side or low at the nape of your neck.

▶ **SEE ALSO**
Braided side bun, pages 158–159
Bow bun, pages 150–151

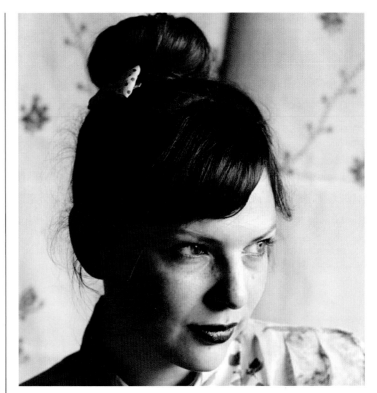

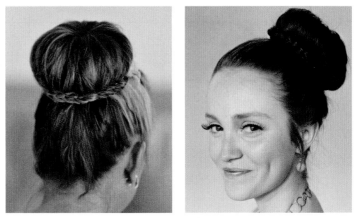

Top: Hairstyling, photography, and modeling by Lana Red Studio.
Bottom left: Hairstyling and photography by Marie-Pierre Sander.
Bottom right: Hairstyling by Ceci Meyer/Tribe Hair Studio, photography by Brittany Lauren Photography.

HOW TO GET IT

WHAT YOU NEED

- Brush
- Strong hair elastic
- Hair donut (optional)
- Small clear hair elastic
- Bobby pins
- Hairspray (optional)

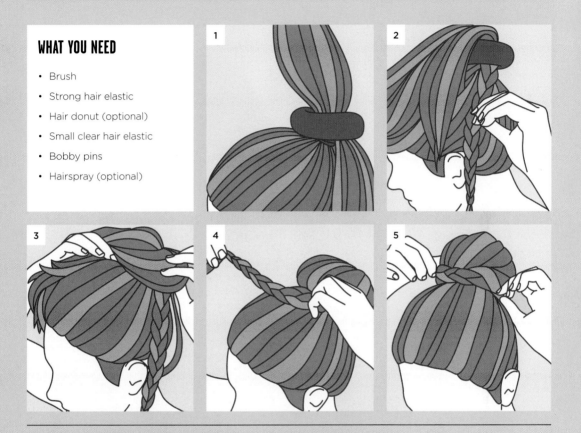

1. Brush your hair and gather it up into a high ponytail. Secure with a strong hair elastic. Separate a section of hair from your ponytail and leave this under the hair donut. Place the donut padding at the base of your ponytail.

2. Split the section of hair under the donut into three and make a basic braid. Secure the end with a small clear hair elastic.

3. Leaving out the braid, make a donut bun (see pages 118–119). If your hair is very long, you can just do a regular top knot bun without the hair donut (see pages 116–117).

4. Pin your bun in place with bobby pins and then curve your braid around the base of your bun and pin with bobby pins.

5. If required, finish with a spritz of hairspray to hold the style and catch any flyaways.

TOP TIP

The thickness of your hair will determine the braid size that's needed to go around the base of your top knot. When you take a section from your ponytail, make sure to leave enough hair to create the bun. You can add in extensions if your hair is fine or too short.

MESSY LOW BUN
THE LOOK

The elegance of this bun lies in its simplicity. There are countless examples of this look being used on the red carpet, and the reason is because it's the perfect style counterpoint to high fashion. The messy low bun sits nonchalantly at the nape of your neck, and creates an aura of effortless perfection, making it an easy everyday style.

DIFFICULTY LEVEL
Easy

IDEAL HAIR LENGTH
Medium to long

HAIR EXTENSIONS NEEDED?
No

ASSISTANCE NEEDED?
No

ACCESSORIES
This undone style is best left without accessories. If you want to go for a bohemian flower power vibe though, add a flower crown or weave flowers into the bun.

TRY THIS
Embrace messy hair! If your hair is curly or wavy, this style is perfect for you. The messy low bun can also be worn to the side for a chic asymmetrical look.

▶ **SEE ALSO**
Low ponytail, pages 24–25
Low pigtail braids, pages 68–69

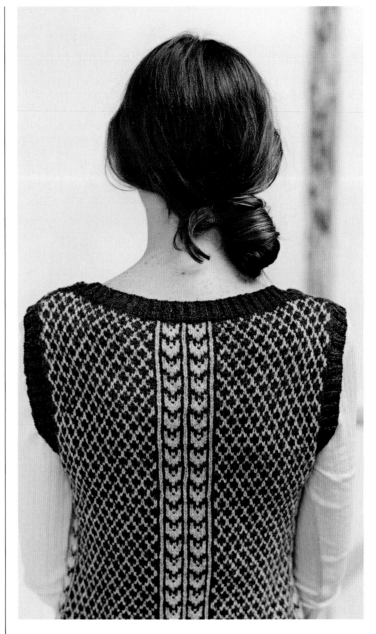

Photograph courtesy of Brooklyn Tweed. Hairstyling by Karen Schaupeter, photography by Jared Flood, modeling by Aine Vonnegut.

HOW TO GET IT

WHAT YOU NEED

- Dry shampoo
- Hair elastic
- Comb
- Bobby pins
- Hairpins (optional)

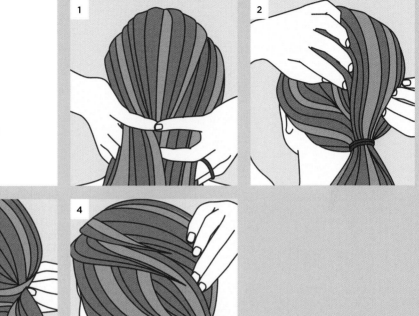

1. Encourage the texture in your hair by using dry shampoo to add texture and body. Don't brush your hair. Instead, use your fingertips to gather your hair into a low ponytail above the nape of your neck, and secure with a hair elastic.

2. Gently backcomb your ponytail to increase the volume in your hair and to make it messier. Pull at the hair above your ponytail so that it's not too tight, and leave some strands loose.

3. Gently twist your ponytail and curve it around its own base to form a bun. Use bobby pins to secure the bun in place. If your hair is thick or curly, try using hairpins for a stronger hold.

4. Pull some pieces of hair from the bun loose so that the bun is uneven. Remember, this is a messy bun, so have some fun with your hair!

TOP TIP

If your hair is freshly washed, you can fake messy hair by using dry shampoo or styling powder to add matte texture. Remember, this style is meant to be imperfect and will look a little different each time you style it.

GIBSON ROLL
THE LOOK

The Gibson roll is an elegant twisted upstyle that's perfect for more formal events. This classic hairstyle became popular in the 1940s and this version is a modern twist on the original design. You'll start with a ponytail and simply roll your hair into a space above it. Gibson rolls are surprisingly simple to do and create an elegant silhouette, with the roll curving around from the back of your neck.

DIFFICULTY LEVEL
Medium

IDEAL HAIR LENGTH
Medium to long

HAIR EXTENSIONS NEEDED?
No

ASSISTANCE NEEDED?
No

ACCESSORIES
This sophisticated hairstyle creates the perfect space for accessories. Add your favorite jewels to the top of the roll to create a refined formal updo. Fresh or silk flowers are also perfect in this chic upstyle.

TRY THIS
You can create a more asymmetrical look by tucking your hair into the Gibson roll off to one side. Create more detail at the sides by leaving the front sections of your hair loose and twisting them back into the top of the Gibson roll.

▶ **SEE ALSO**
Pretzel braid, pages 112–113
Rope bun, pages 164–165

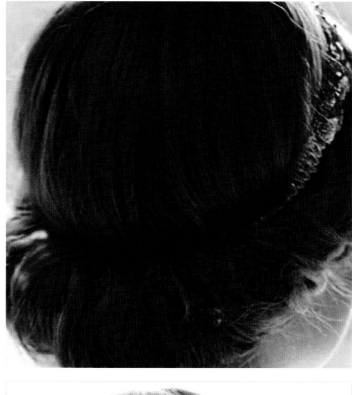

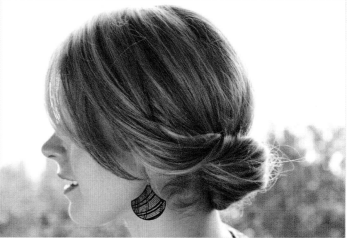

Top: Hairstyling, photography, and modeling by Lana Red Studio.
Bottom: Hairstyling and modeling by Christina Butcher, photography by Xiaohan Shen.

HOW TO GET IT

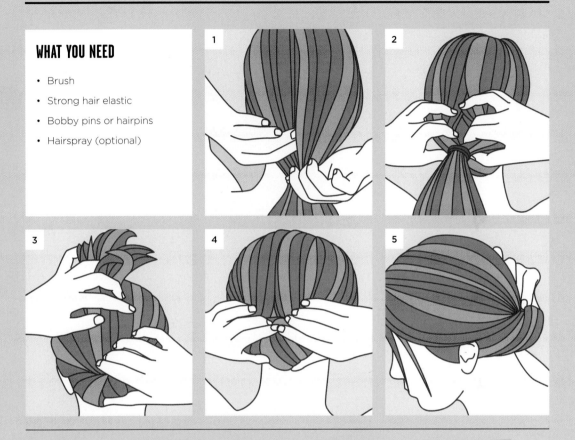

WHAT YOU NEED

- Brush
- Strong hair elastic
- Bobby pins or hairpins
- Hairspray (optional)

1. Brush your hair and gather it into a ponytail that sits low at the back of your head. Secure in place with a strong hair elastic.

2. Next, slide the hair elastic 1 to 2 inches down your ponytail so that you create a space between your hair elastic and your scalp.

3. Push your fingers in above your hair elastic to make a gap. Don't push all the way through; just create a space inside that can hold your hair.

4. Twist your ponytail up and begin pushing it down into this little space. Continue tucking and rolling your ponytail into the gap.

5. Once you have all your hair hidden and tucked away, pin it in place with bobby pins or hairpins. Finish with a spritz of hairspray to hold this hairstyle all day and all night!

TOP TIP

Don't forget to pin the sides of your hair into the roll as well. When you first begin tucking your hair into the space above your ponytail, it may seem tight, but keep twisting your hair to create the roll shape.

FRENCH TWIST
THE LOOK

This classic hairstyle has been worn by style icons for generations. The French twist, roll, or pleat is a chic updo that's as easy as twist and pin! The French twist is a sophisticated hairstyle that works from day to night.

DIFFICULTY LEVEL
Medium

IDEAL HAIR LENGTH
Medium to long

HAIR EXTENSIONS NEEDED?
No

ASSISTANCE NEEDED?
Yes, but you can do this style in your own hair with practice.

ACCESSORIES
The side of the French twist can take any accessory to match your outfit. Try jeweled pins or pin fresh or silk flowers to add a bohemian twist.

TRY THIS
This sophisticated style can be worn sleek and smooth for an elegant evening style, or left loose and messy for a chic daytime style. The French twist is normally worn straight up the back of your head, but it can also be swept to the side for an asymmetrical twist.

▶ **SEE ALSO**
French braid, pages 42–43
Twist and pin bun, pages 142–143

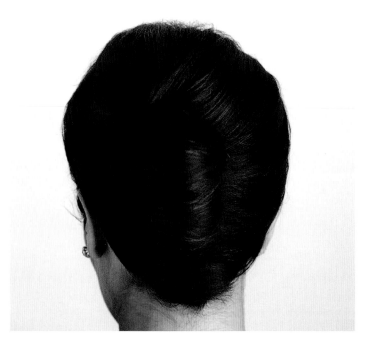

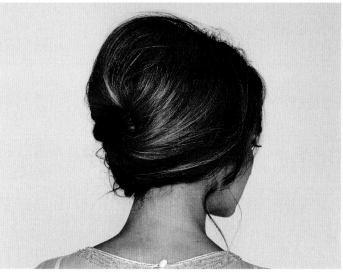

Top: Hairstyling by Ky Wilson/Electric Hairdressing London, photography by Matt Jones Photography.
Bottom: Hairstyling and modeling by Jordan Byers, photography by Tec Petaja.

HOW TO GET IT

WHAT YOU NEED

- Brush
- Bobby pins
- Hairpins (optional)

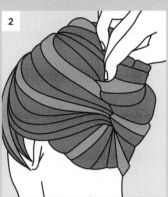

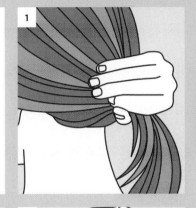

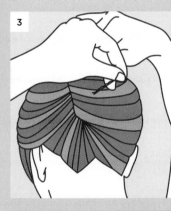

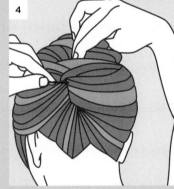

1. Brush your hair and gather it into a low ponytail.

2. Twist the length of your ponytail down and then flip it vertically up.

3. Fold the end of your ponytail over and tuck the ends inside to form a roll.

4. Pin the edge of the twist in place with bobby pins. If you have thick hair, use hairpins for a stronger, more secure finish.

TOP TIP

To keep the French twist in place, angle your bobby pins horizontally. For a secure finish, pin from left to right, twisting the pin 180 degrees so that you catch hair from the top of the twist, and then push the pin underneath the twist.

CHOPSTICK BUN
THE LOOK

The chopstick bun is a chic upstyle that's perfect for long hair. Chopsticks, or hair sticks, are a really easy way to style your hair, plus, as you're not pulling your hair through a hair elastic or using strong clips, you don't risk damaging or breaking your hair either. Twist or roll your hair up and weave the chopsticks through to keep your bun in place. The chopsticks or hair sticks bring some unexpected fun to your hairstyle.

DIFFICULTY LEVEL
Easy

IDEAL HAIR LENGTH
Medium to long

HAIR EXTENSIONS NEEDED?
No

ASSISTANCE NEEDED?
No

ACCESSORIES
The chopsticks are the accessories in this hairstyle. Chopsticks are available in simple, classic styles, or look for beaded and decorated hair sticks.

TRY THIS
Chopsticks and hair sticks can be used to accessorize any twist or bun. Try adding them to high and low buns or French twists.

▶ **SEE ALSO**
French twist, pages 130–131
Rope bun, pages 164–165

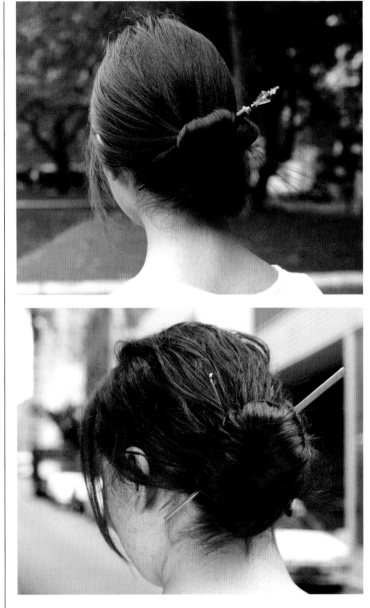

Top: Hairstyling by Christina Butcher, photography by Xiaohan Shen, modeling by Jessica Tran.
Bottom: Hairstyling by Christina Butcher, photography by Xiaohan Shen, modeling by Monica Bowerman.

HOW TO GET IT

WHAT YOU NEED

- Brush
- Chopsticks or hair sticks
- Hair elastic (optional)
- Bobby pins (optional)

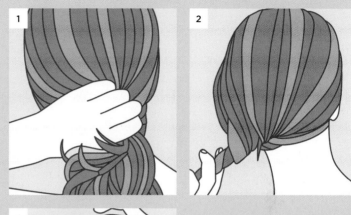

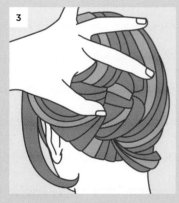

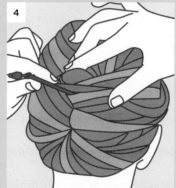

1. Brush your hair and gather it into a low pony.
2. Twist your hair down and then twist up into a pleat (like in a French twist).
3. Tuck the ends of your hair inside the pleat.
4. Push a chopstick or hair stick through to secure the roll. Cross a second chopstick or hair stick through on the other side to hold the bun in place.

TOP TIP

Weave the hair sticks through your bun and the hair underneath to make sure they are secure, and then cross them over to make sure the bun is secure. You can use hair elastics or bobby pins as additional support if you have long or thick hair, but the hair sticks should provide enough hold to your hair.

FIGURE-8 BUN
THE LOOK

The figure-8 bun is, quite literally, a clever twist on the traditional bun. Twisting the hair into a bun and then twisting out the center creates an 8-shaped bun that will set your hairstyle apart from the rest. This is a very neat style that suits professional settings and smart events.

DIFFICULTY LEVEL
Medium

IDEAL HAIR LENGTH
Long

HAIR EXTENSIONS NEEDED?
Yes, this style is best in long to very long hair.

ASSISTANCE NEEDED?
No

ACCESSORIES
Push a decorative hair stick down through the center of the bun to add a little Far Eastern flair to the style.

TRY THIS
Wear your figure-8 bun sideways and turn it into an infinity bun!

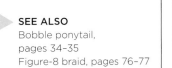
SEE ALSO
Bobble ponytail, pages 34–35
Figure-8 braid, pages 76–77

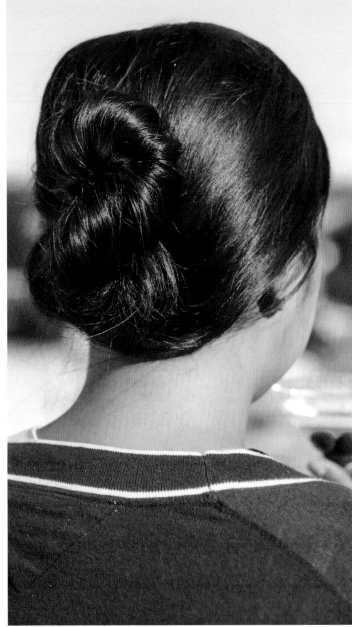

Hairstyling and photography by Christina Butcher, modeling by An Ly.

HOW TO GET IT

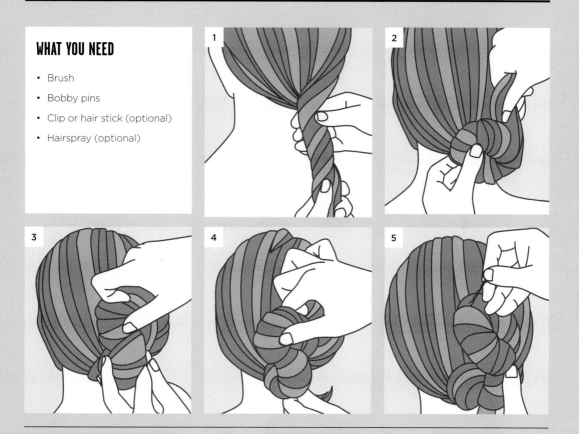

WHAT YOU NEED

- Brush
- Bobby pins
- Clip or hair stick (optional)
- Hairspray (optional)

1. Brush your hair into a low ponytail and twist it down. If you're right-handed, twist counter-clockwise, and if you're left-handed, twist clockwise.

2. Keep twisting your hair around and into a low bun.

3. Take the center part of your bun (the first twist-around) and flip it up and above your original bun.

4. Adjust the twist to sit in a flat figure-8 shape. Ensure the ends are tucked in at the base or side of your bun, depending on how long your hair is.

5. Secure the figure-8 bun with bobby pins at the top and base. You can also insert a hair stick vertically through the center or use a clip across the center to keep this style in place. If needed, use a spritz of hairspray for extra hold.

TOP TIP

Keep the twist tight (but not too tight!) to help maintain the shape and sleekness of this unique bun.

UPSIDE-DOWN BRAID BUN
THE LOOK

Named after its structure, the upside-down braid bun begins as a braid at your neckline and works its way up to a bun at your crown. This style ticks all the boxes in one go: not only does it combine a beautiful braid with a neat, functional bun, it also adds height to your hair and allows for variation. For that reason, this style is great for all occasions, formal, informal, at home, or away on vacation. The only price: practice.

DIFFICULTY LEVEL
Hard

IDEAL HAIR LENGTH
Medium to long

HAIR EXTENSIONS NEEDED?
No, but extensions can be used if you want a big bun to finish.

ASSISTANCE NEEDED?
Yes. The tutorial shows you how to do it in your own hair, but this style is easiest with a partner.

ACCESSORIES
There's a lot going on with this hairstyle, so you really don't need to add anything to it.

TRY THIS
There are so many ways to customize this hairstyle. Try a French braid instead of a Dutch braid at the back. You could even try a French fishtail braid in long hair. Then there's the bun: try a donut bun, a messy bun, or a braided bun!

▶ **SEE ALSO**
French braid, pages 42–43
Top knot with braid, pages 124–125

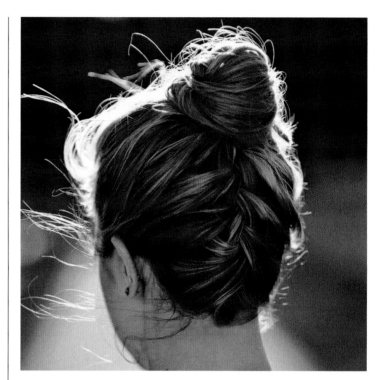

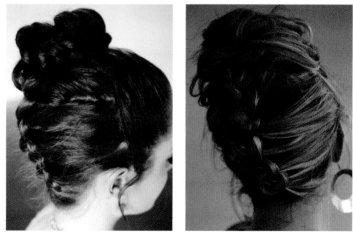

Top: Hairstyling, modeling, and photography by Kayley Heeringa.
Bottom left: Hairstyling by Ceci Meyer/Tribe Hair Studio, photography by Brittany Lauren Photography.
Bottom right: Hairstyling, photography, and modeling by Christina Butcher.

HOW TO GET IT

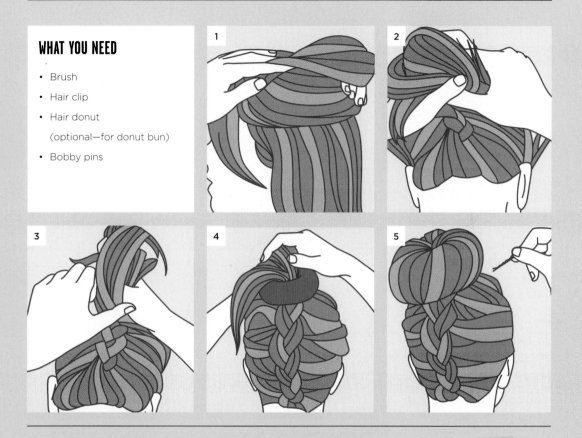

WHAT YOU NEED

- Brush
- Hair clip
- Hair donut
  (optional—for donut bun)
- Bobby pins

1. Brush your hair and clip up the top section of hair above your crown.

2. Hang your head down, ready to begin the braid from the nape of your neck. Take a 1-inch section at your hairline, split it into three, and start to Dutch braid (see pages 44–45).

3. With your head still down, continue braiding in a straight line up the back of your head toward your crown.

4. When you reach your crown, unclip the top section of hair and combine it with your braid in a high ponytail. If you're using a hair donut, place this at the base of your ponytail.

5. Create a donut bun (see pages 118–119). If you have long hair, simply twist your hair around into a top knot and pin in place with bobby pins.

TOP TIP

When your braid reaches the crown of your head, finish in a basic braid so that it stays in place and is easier to combine with the rest of your hair.

MESSY SIDE BUN
THE LOOK

Embrace the shabby chic look and enjoy the freeform shape of this messy side bun. Wear the bun low on your neckline or under your ear for a tighter look. This style creates a soft, relaxed feel, so you'll be comfortable wearing it out with friends or when entertaining. The important thing to remember is there's a big difference between messy and untidy! The key to getting this style right is in the initial stages, when you're forming the bun.

DIFFICULTY LEVEL
Medium

IDEAL HAIR LENGTH
Medium to long

HAIR EXTENSIONS NEEDED?
No, but they can be used to add volume.

ASSISTANCE NEEDED?
No

ACCESSORIES
This simple hairstyle changes with the addition of an accessory. Try incorporating flowers, a diamanté brooch, or a scarf to create different looks.

TRY THIS
Let your bangs or layers hang loose for an even softer look. Alternatively, combine your bangs into the bun to create a low, sweeping, seductive fringe that meets the bun behind your ear.

SEE ALSO
Messy ponytail, pages 32–33
Messy high bun, pages 122–123

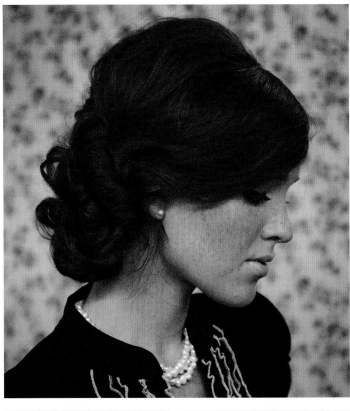

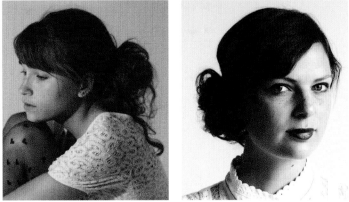

Top: Hairstyling, photography, and modeling by Emily M. Meyers/The Freckled Fox.
Bottom left: Hairstyling, photography, and modeling by Alison Titus.
Bottom right: Hairstyling, photography, and modeling by Lana Red Studio.

HOW TO GET IT

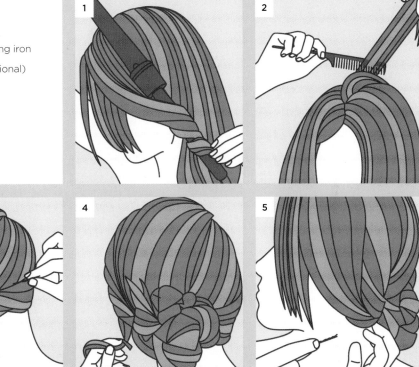

WHAT YOU NEED

- Large-barrel curling iron
- Bristle brush (optional)
- Comb
- Bobby pins
- Hairspray

1. This style looks best with waves or texture in your hair, so use a large-barrel curling iron to curl your hair from the ears down. Break the curls up into waves by running your fingers through or brushing lightly with a bristle brush.

2. Using a comb, tease your hair lightly at the crown to add volume and height to your hair.

3. Twist your hair from the right side of your head around into a low ponytail on the left. Pin the twist in place with bobby pins.

4. Take the rest of your hair and twist and pin up around into a messy bun shape. You can pin your hair in one large bun, or do several smaller buns.

5. Twist and pin any loose layers of hair from the front into the bun and spray with hairspray to set your style in place.

TOP TIP

Remember to keep this style looking messy. If you're having trouble going from ponytail to bun, tie your ponytail with a small elastic first. If backcombing still isn't giving you enough volume, try using extensions or a hair donut, which add amazing volume and are cheap and easy to use.

DOUBLE BUN
THE LOOK

If one bun is fun, a pair makes a pair makes a party, right? Working your hair into this double bun style will give the impression of greater hair volume at the back, while still keeping things under control. This is a sleek yet unusual style that's perfect for the office or a formal dinner. Soften the look by letting your bangs hang loose.

DIFFICULTY LEVEL
Easy

IDEAL HAIR LENGTH
Medium to long

HAIR EXTENSIONS NEEDED?
No

ASSISTANCE NEEDED?
No

ACCESSORIES
A hair stick pushed through both buns would make this style even more unique, and a pretty hair clip on the side of your head would also be an attractive addition.

TRY THIS
For extra quirk, try placing the buns next to one another, or even on a diagonal. You could also try other bun styles, like the twist and pin or sleek bun.

▶ **SEE ALSO**
Mini buns, pages 166–167
Triple twisted bun,
pages 168–169

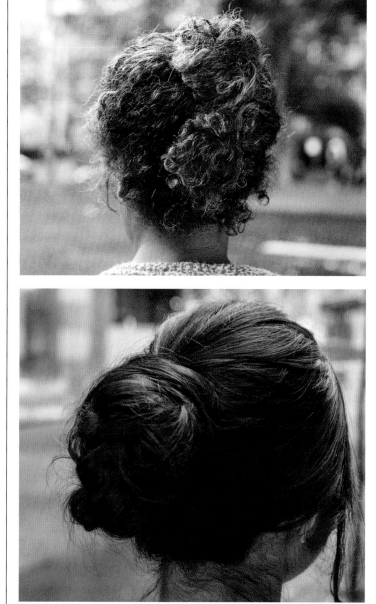

Top: Hairstyling by Christina Butcher, photography by Xiaohan Shen, modeling by Ornella Joaquim.
Bottom: Hairstyling and photography by Christina Butcher, modeling by Arisa Nokubo.

HOW TO GET IT

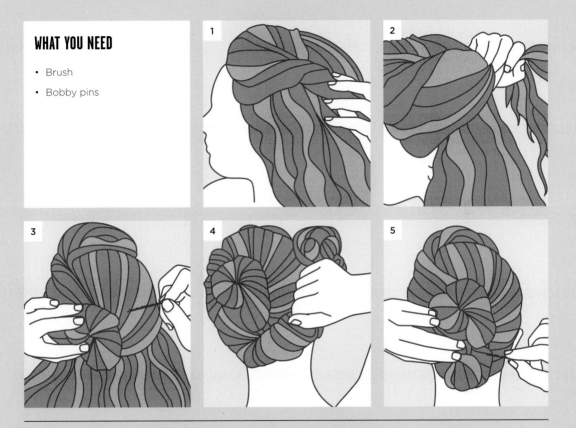

WHAT YOU NEED

- Brush
- Bobby pins

1. Start by brushing your hair and twisting your bangs or front layers off your face and pinning them back with a bobby pin into a small quiff.

2. Combine the quiff with the top section of your hair, taken from above ear level.

3. Twist this top section of hair around and into a bun at the back center of your head. Pin in place with bobby pins.

4. Gather the rest of your hair and twist into a second bun just below the first bun.

5. Pin the second bun in place with bobby pins. Use a few pins to connect the buns and secure them together.

TOP TIP

By pinning the two buns together you not only keep the style looking neat, you also add structure and strength to the buns themselves. Pin through the middle of the top bun and down into the bottom bun, or pin sideways and diagonally through the two. And remember: double the bun, double the fun!

TWIST AND PIN BUN
THE LOOK

The beauty of the twist and pin bun is that it looks really complicated and intricate, but in reality is an easy, simple, and fast style to create. Because this is such a unique, stylish look, you can wear this bun anywhere with ease. Another lazy timesaving style trick is that the twist and pin bun is perfect in dirty hair, as it holds the twists better.

DIFFICULTY LEVEL
Easy

IDEAL HAIR LENGTH
Medium to long

HAIR EXTENSIONS NEEDED?
No

ASSISTANCE NEEDED?
No

ACCESSORIES
Because this is such an intricate style, you won't need to add much to it. However, for more color distinction, you could try a non-permanent balayage effect in your hair, which would give a great color vibe to your style.

TRY THIS
If you have thick hair, try making two buns—much like the double bun (see pages 140–141)—but instead, twist and pin the style in place. If you have long hair, try twisting in smaller sections. The twists will be tighter, and therefore easier to pin. If you have short hair, don't worry about too much twisting, just pin small sections to cover your hair elastic.

▶ **SEE ALSO**
Twist-over ponytail, pages 28–29
Asymmetric chignon, pages 162–163

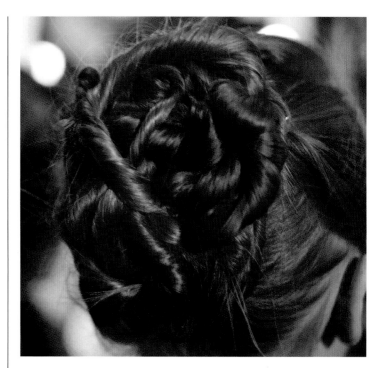

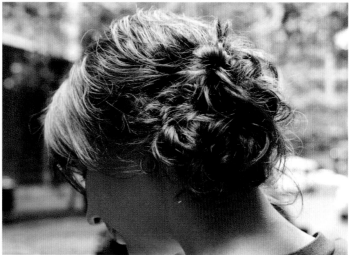

Top: Hairstyling and photography by Christina Butcher, modeling by Olivia English.
Bottom: Hairstyling by Christina Butcher, photography by Xiaohan Shen, modeling by Abigail Schiavello.

HOW TO GET IT

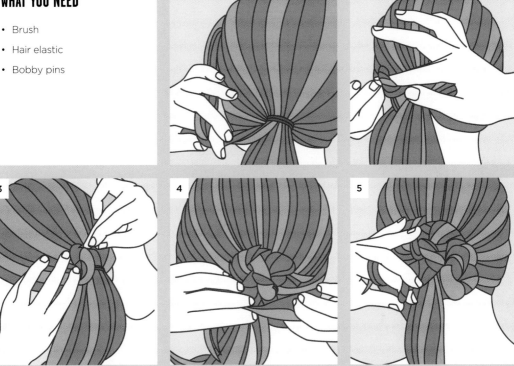

WHAT YOU NEED

- Brush
- Hair elastic
- Bobby pins

1. Part your hair to the side, or wherever your natural part falls. Gently brush or pull your hair back into a ponytail and secure with an elastic.

2. Have a few bobby pins at the ready and start by taking a small section of your ponytail and begin to twist it.

3. Keep twisting this section around your finger again and again until it begins to spring and pull inward toward your head. Allow the lock of hair to fold in on itself and continue twisting into a little knot shape at the base of your ponytail, and then pin in place with bobby pins.

4. Continue with the rest of your ponytail, ensuring that you cover the hair elastic.

5. Leave a section in the center of the ponytail till last. Twist and pin this in the center of the ponytail so that it sits on top of the other sections.

TOP TIP

Work your twists around the outside of the pony; this will ensure you take consistent sections for each twist. Twist the hair around your index finger like a corkscrew. This is the easiest and quickest way to achieve this style. Cross your bobby pins over for a secure finish.

SLEEK BUN
THE LOOK

Neatness is the very essence of the sleek bun. While creating the bun itself isn't too difficult, keeping the rest of your hair and the bun perfect, with as few loose hairs as possible, can be! The sleek bun is a simple yet elegant style and says professional all the way.

DIFFICULTY LEVEL
Easy to medium

IDEAL HAIR LENGTH
Medium to long

HAIR EXTENSIONS NEEDED?
No

ASSISTANCE NEEDED?
No

ACCESSORIES
Keeping it simple is key to this bun and very little should be added to it. More important is the product you use: serum will give your hair the gloss that makes this style shine and hairspray will give it the hold.

TRY THIS
This style is designed with the bun sitting at the back of your head, but you could try an asymmetrical look by positioning the bun to the side of your head, behind your ear.

▶ **SEE ALSO**
Low ponytail, pages 24–25
Pillow bun, pages 154–155

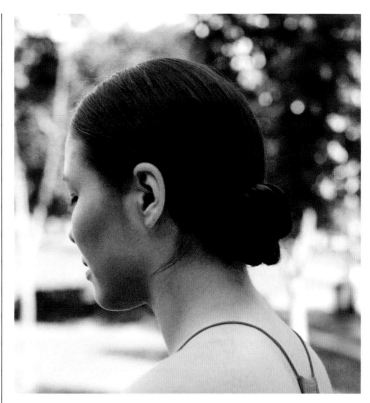

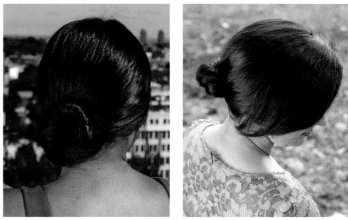

Top: Hairstyling by Christina Butcher, photography by Xiaohan Shen, modeling by Tash Williams.
Bottom left: Hairstyling and photography by Christina Butcher, modeling by Adeline Er.
Bottom right: Hairstyling and photography by Christina Butcher, modeling by Ashleigh Forster.

HOW TO GET IT

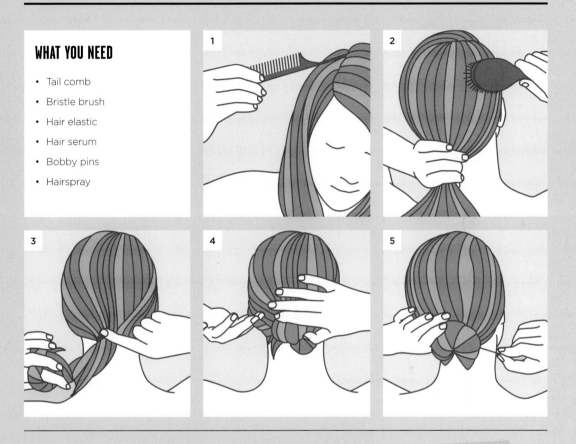

WHAT YOU NEED

- Tail comb
- Bristle brush
- Hair elastic
- Hair serum
- Bobby pins
- Hairspray

1. Use your tail comb to make a neat side part in your hair. You can choose whichever side is best according to your natural part.

2. Brush your hair back into a low ponytail using a bristle brush and secure with a hair elastic.

3. Apply a hair serum to smooth out your ponytail. Move the product down your ponytail and begin to twist your hair down.

4. Keep twisting and circle your hair around the base of your ponytail to form a smooth, tight bun.

5. Secure your sleek bun in place at the sides with bobby pins, and finish with hairspray to catch any flyaways.

TOP TIP

Spray hairspray onto your brush and lightly smooth back your hair to catch even the finest flyaway hairs. Use a fine bristle brush, as this provides the smoothest finish and won't leave brush marks in your hair. This trick holds your hair in place without leaving a helmet-like finish of hairspray.

WATERFALL BUN
THE LOOK

The waterfall braid is one of the most captivating braids, and when woven into a simple side bun it manages to transform a normal bun into an elegant masterpiece. The waterfall sections of this style combine into the bun to create a soft, yet chic, effect. The waterfall bun is a stunning hairstyle for a wedding or formal occasion.

DIFFICULTY LEVEL
Difficult

IDEAL HAIR LENGTH
Medium

HAIR EXTENSIONS NEEDED?
No

ASSISTANCE NEEDED?
Yes, but you can do this style in your own hair with practice.

ACCESSORIES
Create a focus on the side bun with a flower corsage or your favorite jeweled hair clip.

TRY THIS
For long hair, braid the ponytail and pin it round into a braided bun. This style also works well in shorter hair and you can either do a short ponytail or fold the ends over into a small chignon.

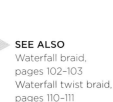

SEE ALSO
Waterfall braid,
pages 102–103
Waterfall twist braid,
pages 110–111

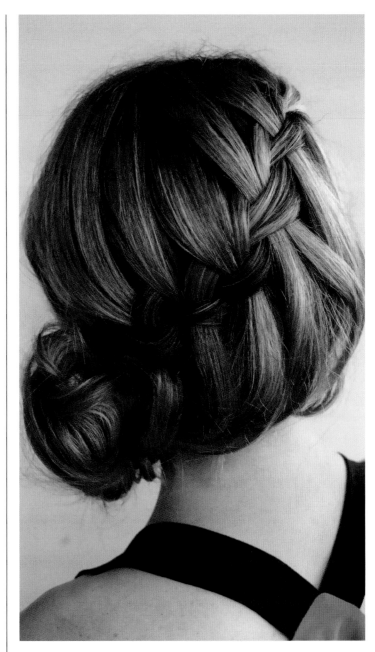

Hairstyling, photography, and modeling by Christina Butcher.

HOW TO GET IT

WHAT YOU NEED

- Brush
- Hair elastic
- Bobby pins
- Comb

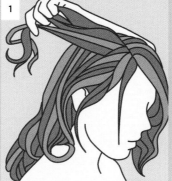

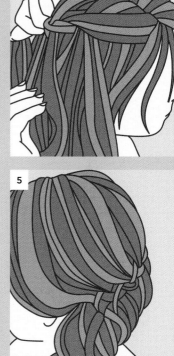

1. Brush your hair and part it. Starting on the right-hand side, take a 1-inch section and split it into three.

2. Start forming a waterfall braid (full instructions on how to do a waterfall braid are on pages 102–103).

3. Once you've reached the lower left side, pull your hair into a ponytail and secure with an elastic, but leave the waterfall sections loose.

4. Scoop up the waterfall sections and twist them into the ponytail.

5. If you have any shorter layers on the first few waterfall sections, use bobby pins to secure them in place. Gently tease or backcomb the ponytail and pin into a messy bun.

TOP TIP

Angle the braid diagonally from the top right of your head down toward the lower left side. You can stretch out your waterfall braid and pull it down to make it appear more diagonal. This style looks great with larger sections, as shown here, or you could do a very fine waterfall braid across as well.

COILED BUN
THE LOOK

Inspired by the Topsy Tail hair tool, this style creates an intricate mess of twists and swirls in a bun that sits low on your head or at your neckline. The process of turning the hair inside itself over and over gives the impression of many buns combined into one. This style can be made to look as messy or as neat as you'd like.

DIFFICULTY LEVEL
Medium

IDEAL HAIR LENGTH
Long

HAIR EXTENSIONS NEEDED?
Yes, you can use extensions for short or fine hair.

ASSISTANCE NEEDED?
No

ACCESSORIES
You can add a clip or flower to the top of the coiled bun. Aside from adding an accessory, this will also help disguise the part at the top of your bun.

TRY THIS
For a different result, try pulling the end of your ponytail through the hole from underneath instead of going up and over. It's slightly more difficult, but it creates a great effect.

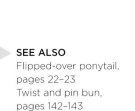

SEE ALSO
Flipped-over ponytail, pages 22–23
Twist and pin bun, pages 142–143

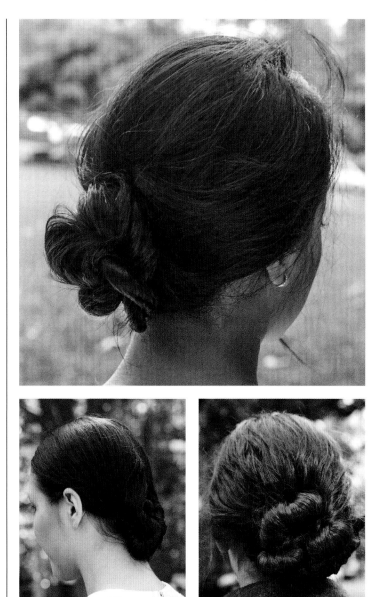

Top: Hairstyling and photography by Christina Butcher, modeling by Patricia Almario.
Bottom left: Hairstyling by Christina Butcher, photography by Xiaohan Shen, modeling by Tash Williams.
Bottom right: Hairstyling by Christina Butcher, photography by Xiaohan Shen, modeling by Monica Bowerman.

HOW TO GET IT

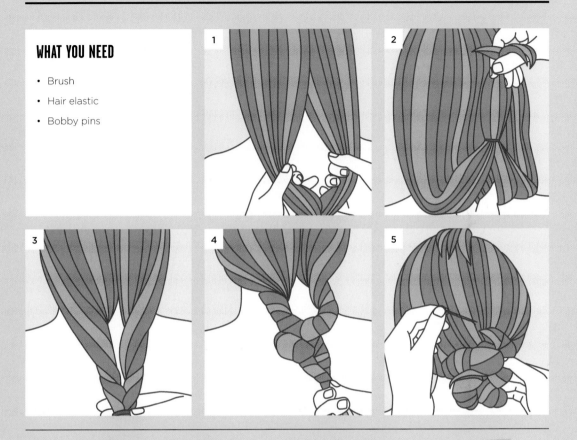

WHAT YOU NEED

- Brush
- Hair elastic
- Bobby pins

1. Brush your hair back into a low ponytail and secure with a hair elastic. Slide the hair elastic down your ponytail, leaving 2 to 3 inches of hair at the end.

2. Split your hair in the middle above your hair elastic and flip your hair up, over, and through the hole above your ponytail.

3. Repeat step 2, flipping your hair through the hole, and you'll see your hair starting to coil and twist.

4. Continue flipping your hair until it coils tightly and forms a bun shape.

5. Tuck the ends of your ponytail underneath and hide them under the coils. Pin your bun in place with bobby pins.

TOP TIP

Make sure the elastic you use is tight enough to hold the end of your ponytail as you flip and twist. If it's not, your hair will come loose and you'll lose the texture you'll need to create this bun.

BOW BUN
THE LOOK

Lady Gaga loves this style, and it's no wonder, as there's a sense of living art about it. Turning your hair into something you usually accessorize with creates an intriguing look that not only mesmerizes but is also super cute! This fun style is perfect for days when you're feeling whimsical and creative.

DIFFICULTY LEVEL
Medium

IDEAL HAIR LENGTH
Long

HAIR EXTENSIONS NEEDED?
No

ASSISTANCE NEEDED?
No

ACCESSORIES
Accessories aren't needed with this style, but wear with polka dots for the ultimate Minnie Mouse look!

TRY THIS
Make a bow bun with only half your hair for a more textured and relaxed feel, or wear the bun at the nape of your neck to produce a sleek look.

SEE ALSO
Bow braids, pages 56–57
Half-up hair bow, pages 152–153

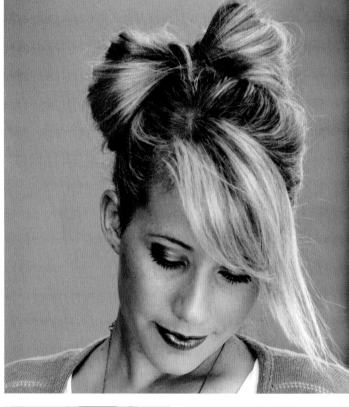

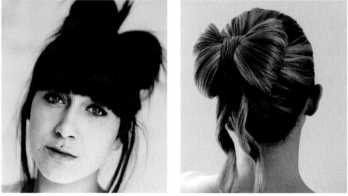

Top: Hairstyling, photography, and modeling by Abby Smith/Twist Me Pretty.
Bottom left: Hairstyling, photography, and modeling by Ana Santl.
Bottom right: Hairstyling, photography, and modeling by Jemma Grace.

HOW TO GET IT

WHAT YOU NEED

- Brush
- Strong hair elastic
- Bobby pins
- Hairspray (optional)

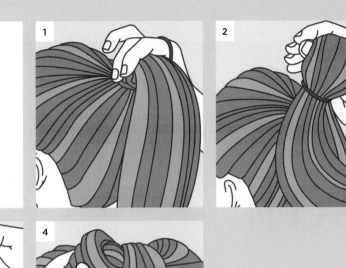

1. Brush your hair up into a high ponytail at the crown of your head. Use a strong hair elastic to secure in place.

2. On the final twist of your elastic, pull your hair only partway through, creating a loop in your ponytail.

3. Split the loop in two and pull each section out and to the side. This will form the sides of your hair bow.

4. Use the tail of your hair to form the center of the bow. Wrap it up and over the middle of the loop and use bobby pins to secure it at the front and back. Adjust the sides of the bow to sit evenly, and use bobby pins to keep them in place. A spritz of hairspray will smooth any flyaway hairs and fix the look.

TOP TIP

Use a bobby pin on either side of the tail that becomes the center ribbon of the bow to keep it straight and in place. If your hair is long, you can tuck the ends of your hair underneath so that they sit inside the loops of the bow.

HALF-UP HAIR BOW
THE LOOK

One of the sweetest, most feminine styles of all, the half-up hair bow takes small sections of hair to create an actual bow with your hair. This delicate look (which is surprisingly long-lasting and stable) is great for picnics, lazy Sunday afternoons, or even a festive holiday party.

DIFFICULTY LEVEL
Easy

IDEAL HAIR LENGTH
Long

HAIR EXTENSIONS NEEDED?
No

ASSISTANCE NEEDED?
No

ACCESSORIES
The hair bow is the accessory to this style, so no further decoration is needed. However, for an extra accent you could run two fine ribbons from the hair elastic to hold the bow in place and thread them around and through the loops.

TRY THIS
Try repeating this style again beneath the original bow to create multiple bows.

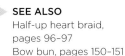

SEE ALSO
Half-up heart braid, pages 96–97
Bow bun, pages 150–151

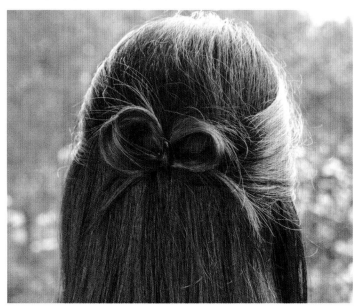

Top: Hairstyling, photography, and modeling by Mindy McKnight.
Bottom: Hairstyling and photography by Christina Butcher, modeling by Carolyn Mach.

HOW TO GET IT

WHAT YOU NEED

- Brush
- Small clear hair elastic
- Bobby pins
- Hairspray (optional)

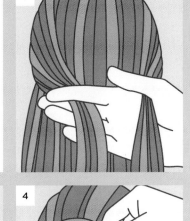

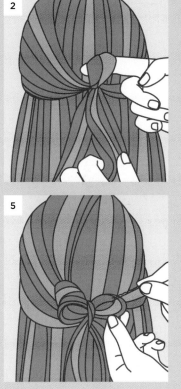

1. Brush your hair and separate two sections of hair, both about 1 inch wide, from each side of your head. Connect these two sections at the back of your head with a small clear hair elastic.

2. Take the elastic around the sectioned hair one more time, but only pull the hair halfway through to form a loop.

3. Split the loop in half and separate the two pieces to form the loops of the hair bow.

4. Take a small piece of hair from the hanging section below the bow and loop it up and around to form the middle of the bow.

5. Secure the bow in place with bobby pins.

TOP TIP

Place your bobby pin horizontally through the center of the bow and pin it to the hair underneath, and pin the loops back to the hair underneath at each side. This allows the style to stay secure and hide your bobby pins at the same time. For extra hold, spray a mist of hairspray.

PILLOW BUN
THE LOOK

This elegant yet restrained chignon is perfect for formal occasions. It's a classic updo, yet the volume you achieve gives this style a sense of adventure. The bun is designed to sit flat on your neckline or low on the back of your head, but you can also wear it higher up for more impact.

DIFFICULTY LEVEL
Medium

IDEAL HAIR LENGTH
Medium to long

HAIR EXTENSIONS NEEDED?
No

ASSISTANCE NEEDED?
No

ACCESSORIES
Because this chignon has a large, flat surface area, you have a lot of space to play with. Try adding flowers or an embellished appliqué (available from craft stores) pinned into the bun. Hair sticks or a large brooch would also work well in this updo. If you're wearing this style as a bride, it offers a perfect place to position the veil.

TRY THIS
Depending on how much you backcomb the filler of this chignon, you can create a fuller or tighter pillow bun. A fuller bun would be lovely for a wedding and is easier to accessorize. A tighter bun makes this style more versatile for everyday wear, such as going to work.

▶ **SEE ALSO**
Pretzel braid, pages 112–113
Gibson roll, pages 128–129

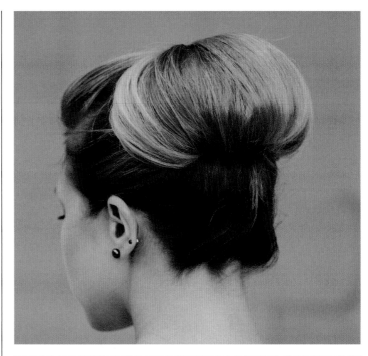

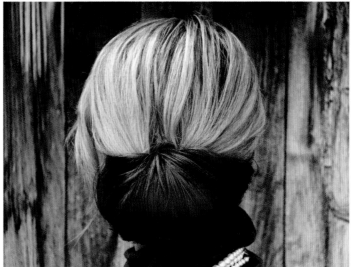

Top: Hairstyling, photography, and modeling by Kayley Heeringa.
Bottom: Hairstyling, photography, and modeling by Abby Smith/Twist Me Pretty.

HOW TO GET IT

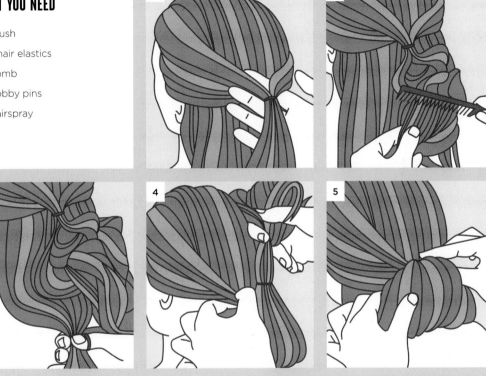

WHAT YOU NEED

- Brush
- 2 hair elastics
- Comb
- Bobby pins
- Hairspray

1. Brush your hair and make a half ponytail by gathering a section of hair from either side of your head. Secure with a hair elastic and leave a gap in the center of your hair.

2. Backcomb your half ponytail. This will create the volume and "stuffing" for the inside of your pillow bun.

3. Gather the rest of your hair into a low ponytail. Secure it with a hair elastic a few inches from the ends of your hair.

4. Bring the lower ponytail up and thread it through the gap in the half ponytail, then tuck it into the gap in the center of the low ponytail.

5. Fan your hair out to form the chignon and tuck the ends of your hair inside the bun. Check that the chignon is even and secure with bobby pins at the top and sides. Finish with hairspray to hold this style in place.

TOP TIP

Use a little hairspray on your comb when you tease your ponytail to make sure the volume stays. Use a stronghold hairspray, but make sure it's one that dries matte. Also check the proportions of your chignon from as many angles as possible when you're fanning out the bun (step 5).

BALLERINA BUN
THE LOOK

This classic ballerina bun has a clean, tight look. The bun swirls all your hair up onto the crown of your head and should hold in place while you pirouette across the dance floor or waltz around productively at work. If ballerinas can pull off this bun, you know it will look elegant and longlasting in your hair too.

DIFFICULTY LEVEL
Medium

IDEAL HAIR LENGTH
Medium to long

HAIR EXTENSIONS NEEDED?
No

ASSISTANCE NEEDED?
No

ACCESSORIES
A tutu? YES! Or . . . pretty up this already sleek, chic chignon with a light ribbon tied around the base of the bun.

TRY THIS
The ballerina bun is traditionally worn on the crown of your head, though you can also wear it at the back of your head or low at the nape of your neck.

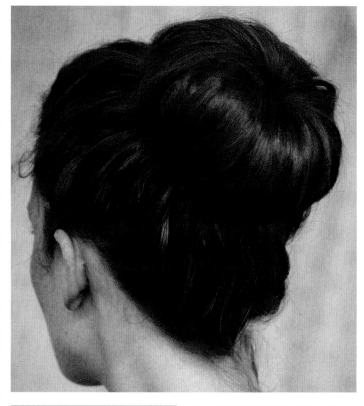

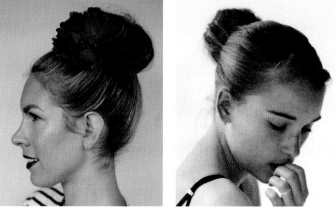

► **SEE ALSO**
Wrapped ponytail, pages 16–17
Chopstick bun, pages 132–133

Top: Hairstyling, photography, and modeling by Emily M. Meyers/The Freckled Fox.
Bottom left: Hairstyling, photography, and modeling by Christina Butcher.
Bottom right: Hairstyling, photography, and modeling by Alison Titus.

HOW TO GET IT

WHAT YOU NEED

- Brush
- Strong hair elastic
- Hair donut
- Clear hair elastic
- Bobby pins
- Hairspray (optional)

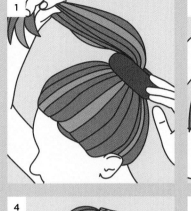

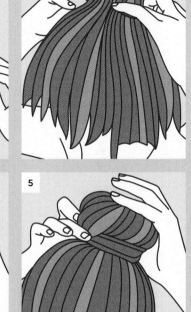

1. Brush your hair into a neat high ponytail that sits on your crown and secure with a strong hair elastic. Place the hair donut at the base of your ponytail.

2. Fan your ponytail out in all directions to cover your hair donut. It helps if you tilt your head forward and look down. Take your clear hair elastic and place it around your hair donut.

3. Ensure your hair donut is completely covered with hair and tighten the clear elastic around the base of the donut, creating the bun shape. If your hair is long, you can lift the donut slightly to allow space underneath for your hair to fit.

4. Holding your bun in place with one hand, carefully twist the rest of your hair around the base of the bun.

5. Pin your ballerina bun neatly in place with bobby pins. A spritz of hairspray will help keep it looking ballet-perfect.

TOP TIP

If your hair is very straight, curl the ends under before you begin to ensure you don't have any pieces sticking out. Also, remember to choose a hair donut that matches the color of your hair.

BRAIDED SIDE BUN
THE LOOK

A simple donut bun can easily be transformed with a side braid detail. In this style a Dutch braid frames your face and wraps around your bun to create a chic look from every angle. The braided side bun can be messed up for a relaxed daytime feel or dressed up for a formal evening event. This type of hairstyle is especially perfect for parties, as you know it's going to last all night.

DIFFICULTY LEVEL
Medium

IDEAL HAIR LENGTH
Long

HAIR EXTENSIONS NEEDED?
No

ASSISTANCE NEEDED?
Yes, but you can do this style in your own hair with practice.

ACCESSORIES
The braid stars as the accessory in this style, although a sparkly pin or flower corsage would also sit beautifully with this bun.

TRY THIS
If you've yet to master the Dutch braid (see pages 44–45), you can do a regular braid and wrap this around the bun to achieve a similar look. If your hair is very long, you can skip the donut bun and just twist your hair into a sleek bun at the side.

SEE ALSO
Mermaid braid, pages 62–63
Fishtail chignon, pages 160–161

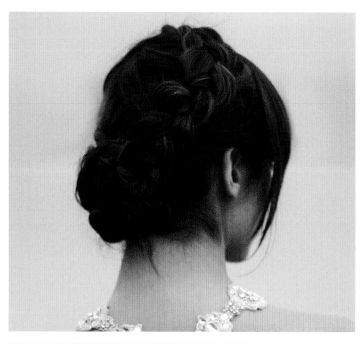

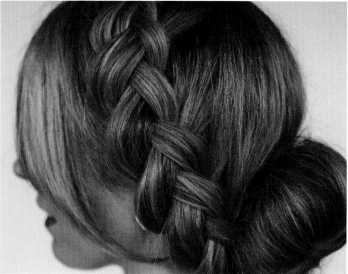

Top: Hairstyling and makeup by Amber Rose, photography by Autumn Wilson Photography, modeling by Laura.
Bottom: Hairstyling, photography, and modeling by Christina Butcher.

HOW TO GET IT

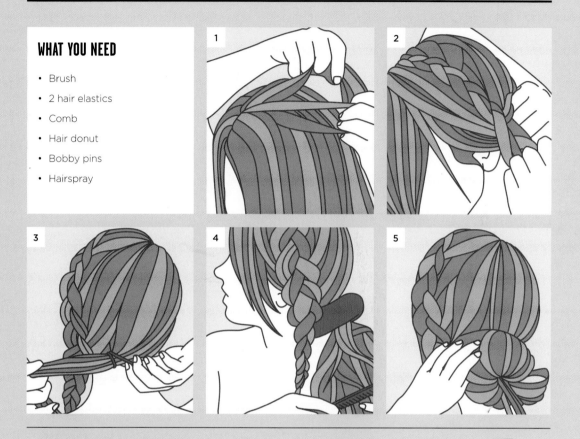

WHAT YOU NEED

- Brush
- 2 hair elastics
- Comb
- Hair donut
- Bobby pins
- Hairspray

1. Start by making a deep side part and brush your hair to remove any knots. Take a 1-inch section on top of your part and split it into three sections. This is the start of the Dutch braid.

2. Cross the right piece under the middle, then the left piece under the right, forming a braid. When you cross the middle section under, add in some hair.

3. Continue braiding, only adding in hair on the right-hand side. Angle your braid along your hairline and over the top of your ear. Stop adding in hair when you pass your ear. Finish the braid and secure with a small clear elastic. Gather the rest of your hair into a side ponytail, next to your braid, and secure with a hair elastic.

4. Backcomb your ponytail and use a hair donut at the base of your ponytail to create a large side bun.

5. Wrap your braid around the base of your bun and pin in place. Add a spritz of hairspray to finish the look.

TOP TIP

To achieve a big, dramatic braid, you'll need to gently pull at the sides to widen it. If you have bangs, you can leave them out or incorporate them. If you leave them out and then change your mind, you can easily pin them back underneath your braid.

FISHTAIL CHIGNON
THE LOOK

This is an interesting twist on the fishtail braid. Sometimes referred to as a seashell braid, this curving fishtail has a shell-like quality and is a beautiful upstyle for day or night. This style is complicated and is one of the harder looks to master, but the effects are stunning and well worth the practice.

DIFFICULTY LEVEL
Hard

IDEAL HAIR LENGTH
Medium to long

HAIR EXTENSIONS NEEDED?
No

ASSISTANCE NEEDED?
Yes

ACCESSORIES
Jeweled pins or a beautiful brooch pinned into the chignon would certainly set this style on fire.

TRY THIS
If you have long hair, you can finish at step 5 and leave your hair out in a side fishtail braid. A simpler version is to do a regular fishtail braid and twist it up into a bun, or make it more complicated by doing a tighter braid and adding in another turn to the braid to create an S shape at the back of your head.

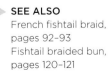

SEE ALSO
French fishtail braid, pages 92–93
Fishtail braided bun, pages 120–121

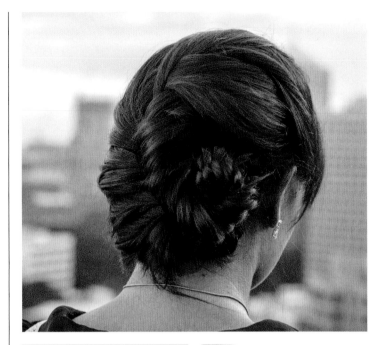

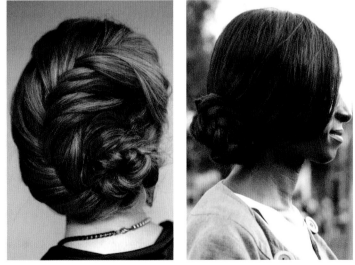

Top: Hairstyling and photography by Christina Butcher, modeling by Elly Hanson.
Bottom left: Hairstyling, photography, and modeling by Christina Butcher.
Bottom right: Hairstyling by Christina Butcher, photography by Xiaohan Shen, modeling by Deauvanné.

HOW TO GET IT

WHAT YOU NEED

- Brush
- Clear hair elastic
- Bobby pins
- Hairspray (optional)

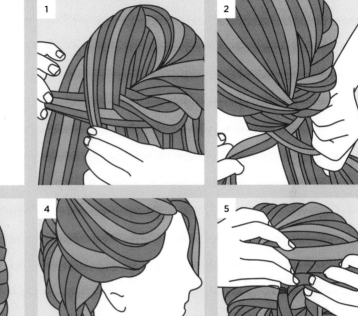

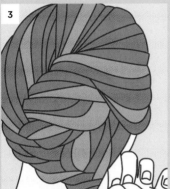

1. Brush your hair back to remove any knots and then make a short part on the right side of your head. Take a section of hair to begin your braid.

2. Make a French fishtail braid from the top right of your head to the bottom left. French fishtail braids use the same technique as a regular fishtail, but you add in extra hair from each side as you braid. To do this, pick up a small section of hair from the left and cross it into your right hand, then pick up a small section of hair on the right and cross it over into your left hand. Repeat this as you braid diagonally downward.

3. When your braid reaches behind your left ear, start to curve it around and then braid along your lower hairline.

4. When you have reached the bottom right side of your head, continue into a regular side fishtail braid until all your hair is braided, and secure the end with a clear elastic.

5. Twist the braid up and around into a spiral bun. Pin in place with bobby pins and spritz some hairspray for extra hold.

TOP TIP

This hairstyle is best in long hair without too many layers. Try to keep each section you add in to the braid small and even. This will emphasize the seashell shape. See tips for mastering the French fishtail braid on pages 92-93.

ASYMMETRIC CHIGNON
THE LOOK

This bun uses a similar technique to the twist and pin to create a fun, asymmetrical style. The difference between the two, however, is that this chignon incorporates more portions of hair into the style. It's also asymmetrical, which adds a touch of glamor to the look and gives it an edge that would suit a party, a formal event, or a day at the office.

DIFFICULTY LEVEL
Medium

IDEAL HAIR LENGTH
Medium to long

HAIR EXTENSIONS NEEDED?
No

ASSISTANCE NEEDED?
No

ACCESSORIES
Pin fresh or silk flowers into the twist to bring out the beauty of this unusual and intricate-looking style. This hairstyle is easy to wear under a hat, as you can customize the size of the chignon to fit.

TRY THIS
This style can be varied infinitely. If your hair is long, twist your hair more to create double buns. For shorter hair, you can twist and fold your hair into a messy chignon. If you think your hair is too short, it's not! You can pin hair that's just 2 inches long.

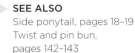

SEE ALSO
Side ponytail, pages 18–19
Twist and pin bun, pages 142–143

Top: Hairstyling by Erin Skipley, photography by Elizabeth Messina, modeling by Faye.
Bottom left: Hairstyling, photography, and modeling by Christina Butcher.
Bottom right: Hairstyling by Christina Butcher, photography by Xiaohan Shen, modeling by Dorothy Jean Joly.

HOW TO GET IT

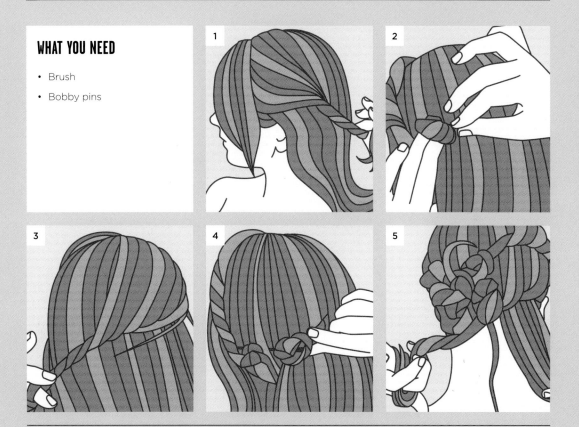

WHAT YOU NEED

- Brush
- Bobby pins

1. Start by twisting a small section of hair from the top left side of your head.

2. Twist the hair tight around your index finger, then twist around the index finger on your other hand to create a small twisted bun on the side of your head. Slide a bobby pin through the twist, pinning it to the hair underneath.

3. Next, twist and pin a small section of hair from the right-hand side of your head, and make a twisted bun next to the first section.

4. Pin the two twists together to create the top of the asymmetrical shape.

5. Keep taking small sections of hair, twist tight around your index finger, then twist around the index finger on your other hand and pin. Continue until all your hair is pinned in place.

TOP TIP

This style looks great when you overlap sections. Weave your bobby pins through more than one twist to create a hairstyle that will hold. You can also cross your bobby pins over each other into an X shape for added hold.

ROPE BUN
THE LOOK

This style adds amazing texture to your look and gives the impression of being far more complicated than it really is. Creating a rope braid in your hair and then twisting it into a bun shape automatically entwines and overlaps your hair. The result is beautiful and intricate and is perfect for weddings or occasions where understated glamor is appreciated.

DIFFICULTY LEVEL
Medium

IDEAL HAIR LENGTH
Long

HAIR EXTENSIONS NEEDED?
No, but a ponytail extension can be used to create a larger bun.

ASSISTANCE NEEDED?
No

ACCESSORIES
You can add flowers, jewels, or even ribbons to the top and sides of the bun to give it an extra accent or to match with your favorite handbag or pair of shoes.

TRY THIS
This technique looks beautiful when combined with the top knot bun (see pages 116–117).

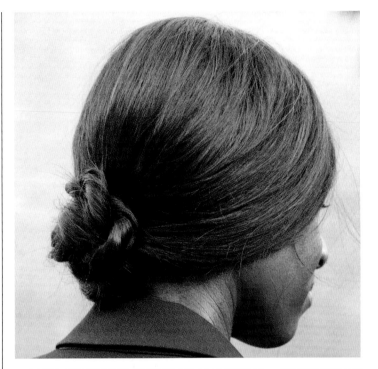

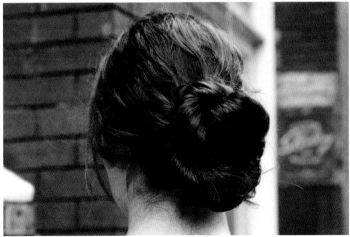

SEE ALSO
Rope twist, pages 94–95
Fishtail braided bun, pages 120–121

Top: Hairstyling by Christina Butcher, photography by Xiaohan Shen, modeling by Deauvanné.
Bottom: Hairstyling by Christina Butcher, photography by Xiaohan Shen, modeling by Monica Bowerman.

HOW TO GET IT

WHAT YOU NEED

- Brush
- Strong hair elastic
- Clear hair elastic
- Bobby pins
- Hairspray (optional)

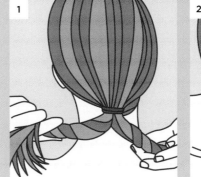

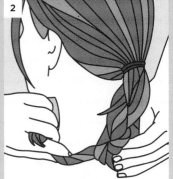

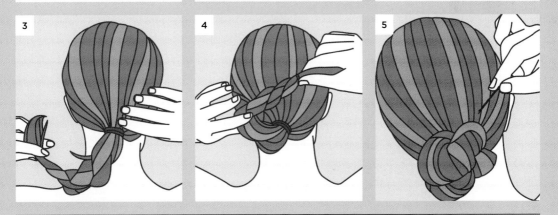

1. Brush your hair back into a low ponytail, secure with a strong elastic, and split your hair into two equal sections.

2. Twist both sections to the left, in a counterclockwise direction.

3. Wind the two sections together, wrapping the left section over the right, and continue to form a rope braid. Remember to twist each section to the left and wrap them to the right. Secure the end of your braid with a clear hair elastic.

4. Bring your braid up and around in a circle to form a bun at the base of your ponytail.

5. Pin in place with bobby pins to secure your bun. Spritz with hairspray for extra hold.

TOP TIP

Use a strong elastic to hold your ponytail in place and a small clear elastic for the end of your braid. This makes the end of your ponytail easier to tuck under the bun. If it's easier, you can twist the sections in a clockwise direction, so long as you wrap them in a counterclockwise direction (see pages 94-95).

MINI BUNS
THE LOOK

If you find the French twist difficult to master, this mini bun hairstyle is the perfect solution. The buns are easier to form without any assistance and will hold your hair well all day long. A row of mini buns down the back of your head in a straight line offers an elegant upstyle with a little edge that works from day to night.

DIFFICULTY LEVEL
Easy

IDEAL HAIR LENGTH
Medium

HAIR EXTENSIONS NEEDED?
No

ASSISTANCE NEEDED?
No

ACCESSORIES
You could pretty this hairstyle up with a jeweled pin, though this style doesn't require much adornment. A ribbon threaded around the buns and tied in a bow at the bottom would be a sweet touch.

TRY THIS
For long hair, braid each section before pinning into a mini bun. You can do as many or as few buns as you like to suit your hair type.

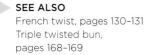

SEE ALSO
French twist, pages 130–131
Triple twisted bun, pages 168–169

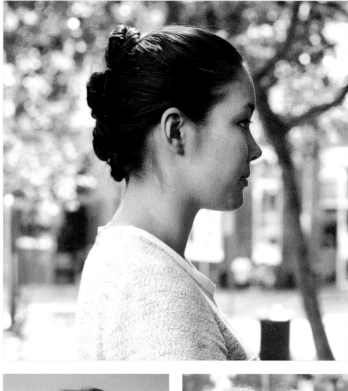

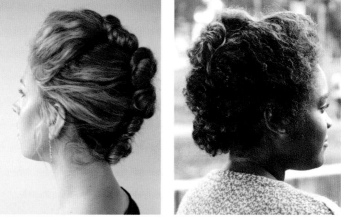

Top: Hairstyling and photography by Christina Butcher, modeling by Tash Williams.
Bottom left: Hairstyling, photography, and modeling by Christina Butcher.
Bottom right: Hairstyling by Christina Butcher, photography by Xiaohan Shen, modeling by Ornella Joaquim.

HOW TO GET IT

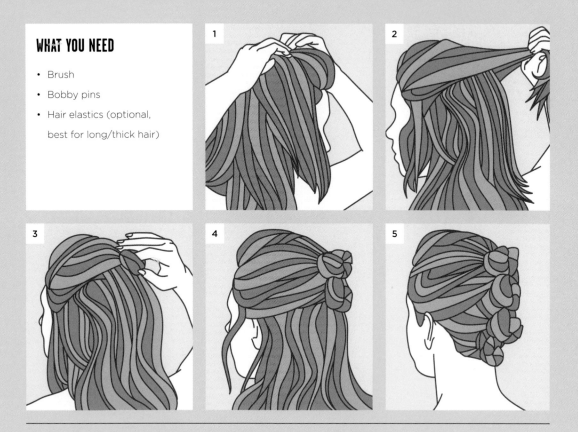

WHAT YOU NEED

- Brush
- Bobby pins
- Hair elastics (optional, best for long/thick hair)

1. Brush your hair and pin back your bangs, or the front section of your hair, then secure with a bobby pin. This style looks good with a little height.

2. Take a small section from each side of your hairline and bring them together into a twist at the back of your head.

3. Twist the section around your finger and pin into a small bun. Secure with bobby pins.

4-5. Repeat steps 2 and 3 until all your hair is twisted and pinned into a line at the back of your head.

TOP TIP

If you have long or thick hair, secure each section in a ponytail with a hair elastic before twisting into a mini bun.

TRIPLE TWISTED BUN
THE LOOK

This is an updo with a twist—three twists, in fact! The triple twisted bun combines the clever trick of twist and pin with a neckline bun style. You can wear this bun as is for a smart, professional look, or accessorize to really make it shine.

DIFFICULTY LEVEL
Easy

IDEAL HAIR LENGTH
Medium to long

HAIR EXTENSIONS NEEDED?
No

ASSISTANCE NEEDED?
No

ACCESSORIES
Pair this style with your favorite headband, or pin flowers in between the buns to create a fresh and relaxed look.

TRY THIS
If you have long or thick hair, why not try four or five buns? A beautiful twist on this style in long hair is to make three braids instead of ponytails and twist them up into a triple twisted braid bun.

▶ **SEE ALSO**
Braided knot buns, pages 62–63
Mini buns, pages 166–167

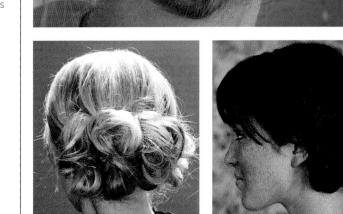

Top: Hairstyling, photography, and modeling by Honor Kristie/Home Heart Craft.
Bottom left: Hairstyling, photography, and modeling by Abby Smith/Twist Me Pretty
Bottom right: Hairstyling, photography, and modeling by Emily M. Meyers/The Freckled Fox.

HOW TO GET IT

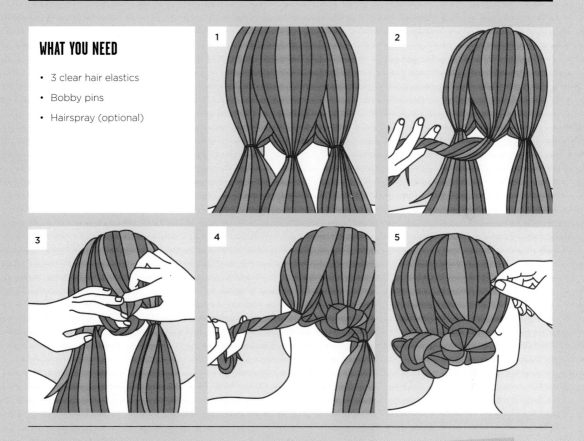

WHAT YOU NEED

- 3 clear hair elastics
- Bobby pins
- Hairspray (optional)

1. Split your hair into three equal sections and secure each one with a clear hair elastic.

2. Start by twisting the middle section down.

3. Wind this twisted section up into a small bun positioned at the nape of your neck. Pin in place with bobby pins.

4. Repeat with the left section, twisting it down and then around to form a bun. Pin in place with bobby pins.

5. Finish with the right section, twisting it down and around to form a bun level with the other two. Pin the style in place with bobby pins. Angle some pins through each bun to pin them together.

TOP TIP

Starting with the middle section first helps you keep the buns level, and pinning them together adds stability. This style works best in second-day hair, although you can always use hairspray for added hold if you have freshly washed hair.

BRAIDED TOP BUN
THE LOOK

The braided top bun is a great way to stand out in a crowd. It's an excellent style if you have long hair and don't quite know what to do with it all. The extra height you get from this style is subtle yet still has a big impact, and for that reason it's perfect for a networking event or if you're out with tall friends!

DIFFICULTY LEVEL
Medium

IDEAL HAIR LENGTH
Long

HAIR EXTENSIONS NEEDED?
No, but you can use a ponytail extension to create a fuller bun.

ASSISTANCE NEEDED?
No

ACCESSORIES
A decorative hairband around the crown of your head will emphasize the bun. A colorful ribbon tied around the base of the bun will also give the style more pizzazz and add extra hold.

TRY THIS
Add a hair donut, as shown in the tutorial, for a giant top bun hairstyle that will make you look taller. You can also do this hairstyle without the extra padding by just twisting your braid around to form a bun.

SEE ALSO
Fishtail braided bun, pages 120–121
Ballerina bun, pages 156–157

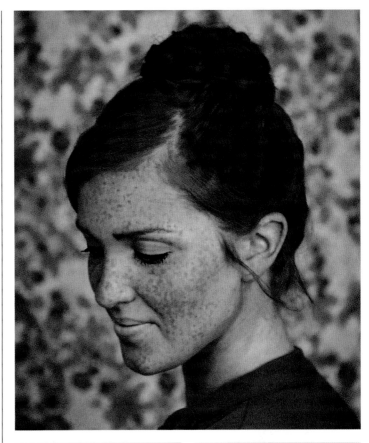

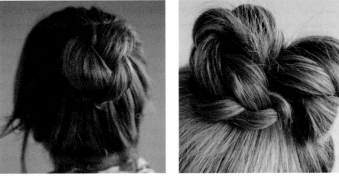

Top: Hairstyling, photography, and modeling by Emily M. Meyers/The Freckled Fox.
Bottom left: Hairstyling, photography, and modeling by Christina Butcher.
Bottom right: Hairstyling, photography, and modeling by Christina Butcher.

HOW TO GET IT

WHAT YOU NEED

- Brush
- Strong hair elastic
- Hair donut
- Clear hair elastic
- Bobby pins
- Hairspray (optional)

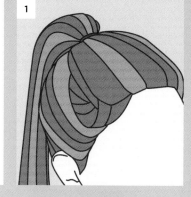

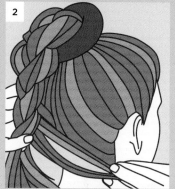

1. Brush all your hair up into a high crown ponytail and secure with a strong elastic.

2. Place a hair donut at the base of your ponytail. Split your ponytail into three and make a basic braid.

3. Braid all the way to the end of your ponytail and secure the end with a small clear hair elastic.

4. Twist your braid around your hair donut to form the braided top bun. Tuck the ends of your braid under and pin in place with bobby pins. Stretch your braid out to emphasize the shape and to make sure the donut is covered. If required, spritz with hairspray for added hold.

TOP TIP

The secret to the perfect high crown ponytail is to brush your hair with your head turned downward. Use one hand to hold your hair at the top of your head and smooth your hair with a brush held in your other hand. Make sure your ponytail is even, then secure with a strong hair elastic.

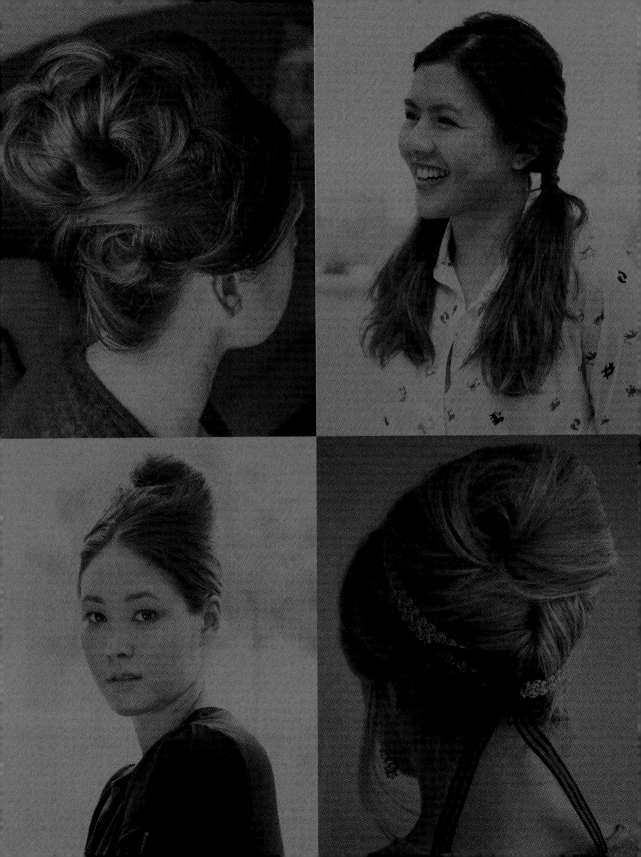

CHAPTER 4
BOUFFANTS

BOUFFANT PIGTAILS
THE LOOK

This is a chic way to wear pigtails—without being mistaken for a little girl! The teased crown creates height and volume, and the twisted back adds detail to low pigtails. This grown-up version of a childhood favorite is great for a day by the beach or for catching up with friends. Audrey Hepburn immortalized this style in 1961 in *Breakfast at Tiffany's*. This movie was the inspiration for all the styles in this chapter, and it popularized the beehive as a major hair trend.

DIFFICULTY LEVEL
Easy

IDEAL HAIR LENGTH
Medium to long

HAIR EXTENSIONS NEEDED?
No

ASSISTANCE NEEDED?
No

ACCESSORIES
A flower or jeweled clip can be pinned at the twist at the back for extra detail. Large sunglasses and breakfast at Tiffany's are a must!

TRY THIS
Audrey wore this style with short bangs, and side-parted front layers are in keeping with the retro style. Braid your pigtails and pin into a chignon at the nape of your neck for a chic upstyle.

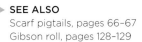
SEE ALSO
Scarf pigtails, pages 66–67
Gibson roll, pages 128–129

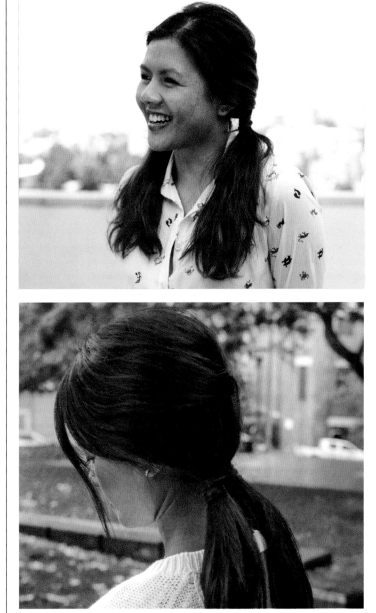

Top: Hairstyling by Christina Butcher, photography by Xiaohan Shen, modeling by Sophia Phan.
Bottom: Hairstyling and photography by Christina Butcher, modeling by Patricia Almario.

HOW TO GET IT

WHAT YOU NEED

- Comb
- Bobby pins
- 2 hair elastics

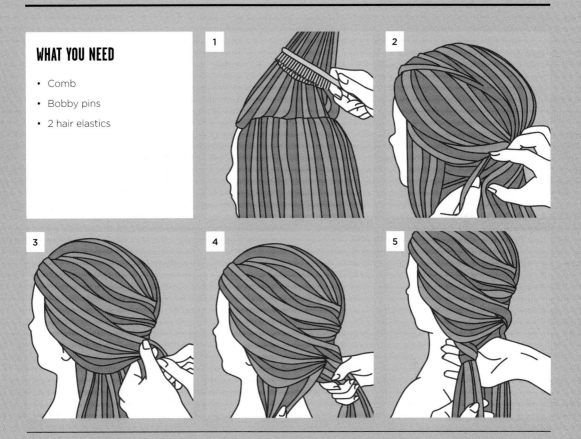

1. Start by backcombing the top section of hair at the crown of your head to create the bouffant shape.

2. Next, gently comb it back and smooth over the top layer of hair.

3. Take a section of hair from above each ear and twist the sections over at the back, and use a bobby pin vertically to pin in place. This will support the bouffant and keep the volume in your hair. Repeat with another twist if necessary.

4. Split your hair into two sections to form the pigtails. Secure each pigtail with an elastic.

5. Take a section of hair from the underside of the pigtail and wrap it around the hair elastic to cover it. Pin in place with a bobby pin underneath.

TOP TIP

Prep your hair for extra volume before starting this style. Wash your hair with a volumizing shampoo and apply mousse to towel-dried hair before blow-drying.

CLASSIC 1960s BOUFFANT
THE LOOK

This is the most chic updo to come out of the 1960s. The beauty of this timeless classic is its stylish versatility. Perfect for a black-tie soirée or an important event, but also a great choice for work, this style's got it covered. Of course, the bouffant is best suited to the vintage '60s look, so think pencil skirts, simple straight dresses, and beautiful earrings. Also known as the beehive, this style originated in the 1950s and became iconic in the 1960s. Celebrities, notably Brigitte Bardot, favored the beehive style and made it extremely popular in the United States, where it was commonly styled using a fork!

DIFFICULTY LEVEL
Medium

IDEAL HAIR LENGTH
Medium to long

HAIR EXTENSIONS NEEDED?
Yes, the more hair the better for this style.

ASSISTANCE NEEDED?
No

ACCESSORIES
A wide satin headband is the perfect hair accessory to finish off the front of your bouffant. For an evening look, add a tiara!

TRY THIS
Leave this style relaxed and messy, with lots of volume at the top. You can modernize the bouffant with subtle volume, or wear your hair half down.

▶ **SEE ALSO**
1960s ponytail, pages 30–31
Gibson roll, pages 128–129

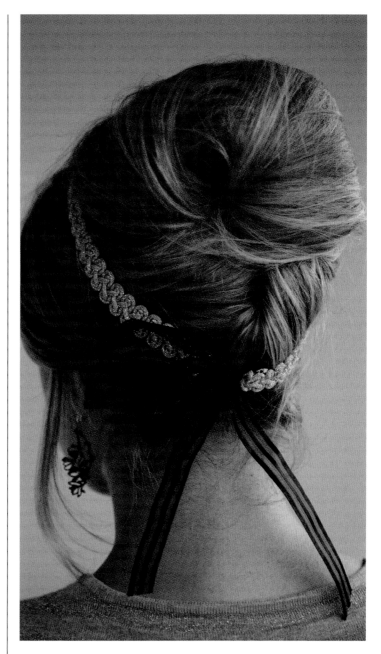

Hairstyling, photography, and modeling by Christina Butcher.

HOW TO GET IT

WHAT YOU NEED

- Hair clip
- Bobby pins or hairpins
- Comb
- Bristle brush
- Hairspray

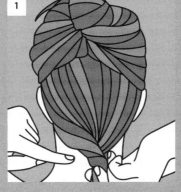

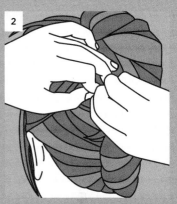

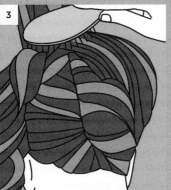

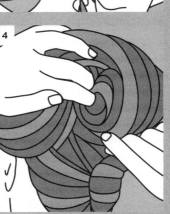

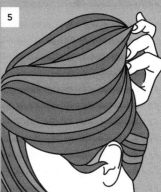

1. Part your hair from ear to ear at the back and clip the top section up. Take the bottom section of hair and twist it to the right into a low pony.

2. Flip your pony up and keep twisting your hair into a French twist (see pages 130–131). Tuck the ends of your hair inside the twist and pin in place with bobby pins.

3. Backcomb the top section. Start at the crown and use a comb or fine bristle brush to tease your hair at the roots until it's almost standing up on its own. Use the fine bristle brush to smooth over the front layer.

4. Roll the ends of the top portion of hair around and under to form the base of your bouffant. Position it above the French twist and pin in place using bobby pins or hairpins.

5. Pin back the sides of your hair and make sure the top of your bouffant is smooth. If you have bangs, you can leave them loose or pin them back by your ear. Finish with lots of hairspray, just like they did in the 1960s. This will help your bouffant last all day and all night!

TOP TIP

To achieve huge volume in the bouffant, you'll need to use product on your hair to add structure and hold. If you have fine or soft hair, apply a volumizing mousse and use a blow-dryer to set it into your hair. If your bouffant isn't holding, just keep backcombing and use more hairspray!

BEEHIVE WITH A BUN
THE LOOK

When the classic 1960s bouffant just isn't big enough, try a beehive with a bun. Using as much hair as possible is key to this style, and the hidden bun gives a more structured hold to the height of your beehive. You'll be ducking under doorways before you know it! This style still has the glamorous, seductive feel of the classic bouffant, just super-charged. This modern take on the beehive goes with my own motto: the higher the hair, the closer to heaven!

DIFFICULTY LEVEL
Hard

IDEAL HAIR LENGTH
Medium to long

HAIR EXTENSIONS NEEDED?
Yes, the more hair the better for this style.

ASSISTANCE NEEDED?
Yes, the tutorial offers a guide for doing this in your own hair, but it is much easier with help.

ACCESSORIES
An upstyle like this calls for statement earrings—the bigger the better.

TRY THIS
This hairstyle is itself a variation on the classic 1960s bouffant, and you can wear it with your hair half up for a more relaxed, messier upstyle.

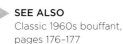

SEE ALSO
Classic 1960s bouffant, pages 176–177

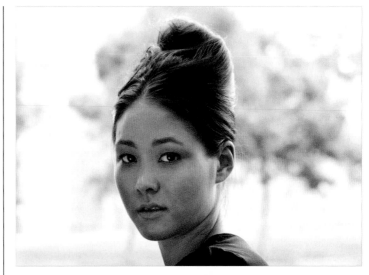

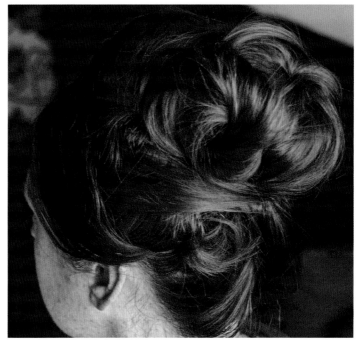

Top: Hairstyling by Christina Butcher, photography by Xiaohan Shen, modeling by Tash Williams.
Bottom: Hairstyling and photography by Christina Butcher, modeling by Monica Richmond.

HOW TO GET IT

WHAT YOU NEED

- Hair clip
- Comb
- Brush
- Bobby pins
- Hair elastic
- Hair donut
- Hairspray

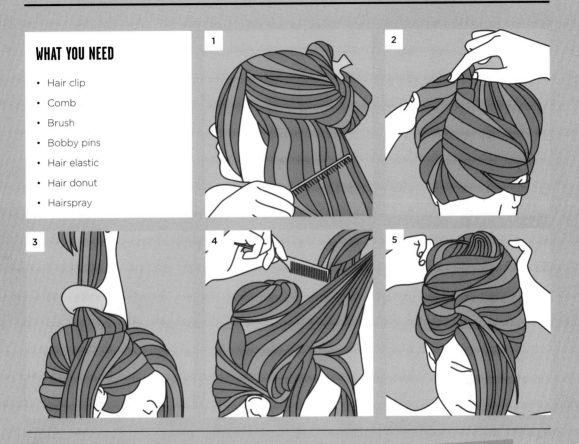

1. Separate your hair from ear to ear and clip the top section up. Use a comb to backcomb the bottom section of your hair at the roots.

2. Twist the bottom section down and then flip it up into a French twist (see pages 130–131). Brush the sides of your hair to smooth it back, tuck the ends of your hair inside the twist, and pin in place with bobby pins.

3. Take a 3-inch section of hair from the top at the crown, but make sure to leave enough hair at the front and sides for the later steps. Secure this section in a ponytail with a hair elastic and place the hair donut at the base. Backcomb your pony and cover the hair donut to create a bun.

4. Backcomb the rest of your loose hair. Focus on teasing at the roots and midlengths to create the shape and volume of the beehive.

5. Smooth back the top of your hair with your comb or brush and position your hair over and around the bun to create your beehive. Pin in place with bobby pins and use lots of hairspray to keep your hairstyle up. If you have bangs, you can leave them out or sweep them back.

TOP TIP

Visualize the style before you start to backcomb. Once the bun is in place, backcomb your hair with the shape in mind. This style adds extra lift, so you can get that wow factor with your super-high beehive even if you have fine or medium-length hair.

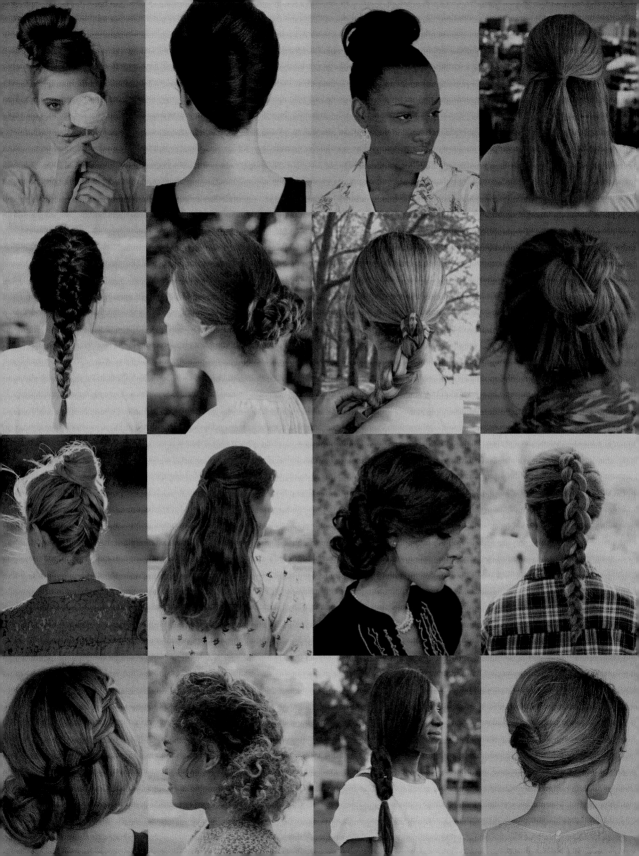

CHAPTER 5

RESOURCES

HAIRSTYLING TOOLS

Blow-dryer

A good blow-dryer is essential for your hairstyling kit. A professional dryer is best and will last a long time. Look for ionic blow-dryers, as this system reduces static and creates less frizz in your hair.

**Curling iron
(without a clamp)**

This newer type of curling wand is becoming increasingly popular. Use a heat-protective glove to protect your hand as you wind your hair around the barrel. This type of iron avoids the dents that a curling iron with a clamp can leave in your hair.

Conical curling iron

Barrel curlers have a set width, so always create the same sized curls. A conical curler allows you to create curls in different sizes and shapes, depending on where on the iron you heat-style your hair.

Diffuser

An attachment for your blow-dryer that disperses the air flow to spread it over a larger area. Use your dryer on a low speed with a diffuser to style curly hair.

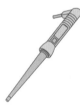

**Curling iron
(with a clamp)**

The original curling wand, which is designed to heat your hair to create curls and waves. The clamp helps you to hold your hair as you wind it around the barrel.

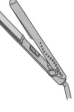

Flat iron

Also known as straighteners or straightening irons, these heat-styling tools make your hair smooth and sleek. The ceramic plates glide down your hair, leaving it straighter than any blow-dryer can. You can also twist the iron through your hair to create waves.

Bristle brush
These brushes are best for smoothing your hair. They are made with boar bristles, which are gentler on hair than plastic brushes. The bristles also distribute your hair's natural oils and encourage shine.

Paddle brush
Great for detangling long hair. You can also use this brush when blow-drying, although it won't give as smooth a finish as a round brush.

Clips
Large clips are perfect for keeping sections of your hair out of the way while you are styling. Use the smaller flat clips to pin up curls when setting your hair.

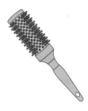

Round brush
Use a round brush to create volume and waves when blow-drying your hair. Wrap the ends of your hair around the brush to create flicks and waves, and use the cool-shot button on your blow-dryer to set the style.

Comb
Use the wide side to de-tangle wet hair and the fine side to backcomb for added height and volume.

Tail comb
Use the tail to section hair and create neat part lines. This fine comb is also great for backcombing and, used with straightening irons, will ensure there are no knots in your hair.

Bobby pins

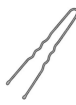

The most important tool for any updo. Bobby pins are very handy, and you should always keep some in your bag. Choose pins that match your hair color, and look for professional pins, which are stronger than generic brands.

Hair donut

This round sponge padding is shaped like a donut and acts like a push up bra for your hair. It gives instant volume and shape to your bun. Hair donuts are available in different colors to match your hair. You can also make your own by cutting the toe off a sock and rolling it into a donut shape.

Fringe pins

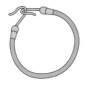

These pins are fantastic for chignon and French twist styles, and even for securing braids in thick hair. The trick is to squeeze the pins a little when inserting them so that they spring into place and provide extra hold when you release them.

Hair elastics

Use to secure ponytails and braids as well as hair sections under buns. Find the right size and strength to hold your hair and look for snag-free elastics without metal connectors. Clear elastics are best for the ends of braids, as they are virtually invisible in your hair. Scrunchies should never be used!

Hair bungees

Rather than pulling your hair through an elastic, hair bungees wrap around your hair. They are adjustable to suit hair thickness and are best for long hair, as they make it easier to secure ponytails. They are also curly-hair friendly—regular elastics can crush curls as you pull the hair through.

Topsy Tail

This plastic tool works like a giant sewing needle for your hair. Place it above your hair elastic and thread your ponytail through the loop to neatly twist your hair back through itself. It's possible to re-create styles like the flipped-over ponytail (see pages 22–23) without it, but the Topsy Tail gives a neater finish.

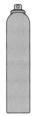

Hairspray

The ultimate finishing spray for when you want your hairstyle to last. Don't overdo it with the hairspray though, as it can make your hair sticky and heavy. Choose a light, flexible hairspray when curling or backcombing your hair, and go for a strong-hold spray to fix an updo in place.

Serum

Serum smooths and adds shine to hair. It's available in tiny bottles, as you need only a drop or two to add gloss over your hair. Remember, a little goes a long way, and too much serum can make your hair look oily.

Styling powder

Styling powder adds instant volume. Lightly sprinkle these fine powders onto the roots of your hair and massage gently with your fingertips for an instant lift. These powders have a matte finish, so you can add more if you need to, and they can refresh oily roots.

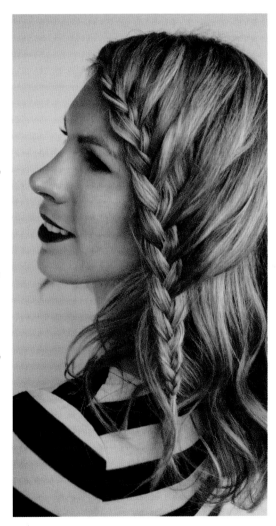

SCHOOLS AND FURTHER EDUCATION

Love styling hair and want to do it every day? You can create a career out of making people look and feel beautiful as a cosmetologist.

Hairdressing is a rewarding career that combines technical skills with a creative, communicative outlet, and offers flexibility and the opportunity to run your own freelance business or salon. You'll also be able find work almost anywhere in the world.

To be a successful hairdresser, you'll need to be a good communicator. Hairdressing is a very social career. When people go to the salon, it's not just their hair that's expecting attention; people go for an experience. You'll have to be a people person, love listening, and be able to keep up with all your clients' lives.

It's important you understand color, shape, and style, and being able to visualize the end result is vital. Styling hair also takes an impressive number of skills in order to become proficient. Everyone's hair is different, so you'll need to be artistic and creative, with a flair for solving problems. On top of this you'll need to be interested in—and good at—following trends, and be on the lookout to start your own.

Most of all, you'll need to love hair, fashion, and style. If you have all these qualities, you'll make one heck of a hair stylist! Good luck!

The licensing requirements to register as a cosmetologist or hairdresser vary by state and country, so it's best to find a school in your local area. Here are some links to follow up if you're interested in pursuing a career as a hairdresser.

North America

Arrojo Cosmetology School (NEW YORK) Arrojocosmetology.com

Aveda Institute (NATIONWIDE AND IN CANADA AND AUSTRALIA) Aveda.edu

Empire Beauty Schools (NATIONWIDE) www.empire.edu

Paul Mitchell Schools (NATIONWIDE) Paulmitchell.edu

Regency Beauty Schools (NATIONWIDE) www.regencybeauty.com

Love hair and just want to find out more ways to style yours? Head online to these sites to discover more about how to look after and style your hair:

www.hairromance.com
www.latest-hairstyles.com
www.cutegirlshairstyles.com
www.princesshairstyles.com
Hairdresser on Fire —
www.hdofblog.com
www.twistmepretty.com
www.hairandmakeupbysteph.com

GLOSSARY

Backbrush
A technique that involves using a brush to tease hair and build volume.

Backcomb
Also known as teasing, ratting, matting, or French lacing. This technique involves combing small sections of hair from the ends toward the scalp, creating a cushion or base for hairstyles that require volume.

Balayage
A highlighting technique where color (typically a lightener) is painted onto hair with a brush. This produces a gradation of color, like a sun-kissed effect, from roots to ends.

Bangs
Also known as a fringe, this is the front section of hair that falls across the face. You can style bangs in lots of ways—blunt bangs, curved bangs, or swept to the side. You can also leave them loose or include them in your hairstyles.

Blow-dry
Also called a blow-out. This is a styling technique where hair is dried and styled with a blow-dryer and usually with a round brush. You can also use a paddle brush when blow-drying long hair.

Braid
Also known as a plait. Chapter 2 in this book is devoted to this versatile styling technique, which involves winding or weaving sections of hair into each other.

Chignon
A twisted bun that usually sits low at the nape of your neck. The word "chignon" comes from the French phrase *chignon du cou*, which means "nape of the neck."

Crown
This is the area of the head along the top and back of the skull.

Curling iron/wand
A round- or conical-barrel heat styling tool that creates curls and waves.

Flat iron
A styling tool that straightens your hair. Also known as a straightening iron.

French plait
The same as a French braid.

Hair elastic
Used to tie up and secure hair. Also known as a hair band or hair tie.

Hair extensions
Additional hair that is attached to your natural hair to add length, volume, or texture. Extensions can be permanently attached with glue or tape or temporarily clipped in.

Hairline
This is the hair that grows along the outermost perimeters of your head, including around the face and ears and along the neck.

Hairspray
Also known as finishing spray, this is a styling product that comes in the form of a mist and is used to set a style in place.

Neckline
The neckline is part of the hairline, but specifically refers to the hair that begins at the back of the neck.

CONTRIBUTORS

Abby Smith, Twist Me Pretty
www.twistmepretty.com

Alison Titus
www.alison.titus.bz

Amber Rose Hair + Makeup
www.amberrosehairandmakeup.com
Photography: Eliesa Johnson Photography
www.eliesajohnson.com
Autumn Wilson Photography
www.autumnwilson.com
Wardrobe: Anne Kristine Lingerie
www.annekristinelingerie.com

Ana Santl
www.iamnotana.com

Bailey Tann
www.baileytann.com

Breanna Rutter, How To Black Hair LLC
www.howtoblackhair.com

Brittany Lauren Photography
www.brittanylauren.net
Hairstyling: Ceci Meyer, Tribe Hair Studio
www.tribehairstudio.com

Brooklyn Tweed
www.brooklyntweed.net
Photography: Jared Flood, www.brooklyntweed.net
Hairstyling: Veronik Avery, www.stdenisyarns.com
Karen Schaupeter, www.karenschaupeter.com
Make-up: Hannah Metz, www.hannahkristinametz.com

Chrissann Gasparro
www.ducksinarowevents.blogspot.com
Photography: Drew Nebrig
www.ducksinarowevents.blogspot.com

Christie Cagle
www.christicagle.com
Photography: Christine Hahn
www.christinehahnphoto.com
Lou Mora, www.loumora.com
Makeup: Jennifer Fiamengo, www.jfmakeup.com

Christina Butcher, Hair Romance
www.hairromance.com
Photography: Xiaohan Shen, www.xiaohan.com.au

Emily Goswick, The Rancher's Daughter
www.egoswick.com
www.egoswick.blogspot.com

Emily M. Meyers, The Freckled Fox
www.freckled-fox.com

Erica Gray Beauty Company
www.ericagray.com

Erin Skipley
www.erinskipley.com
Photography: Elizabeth Messina
www.elizabethmessina.com
Jasmine Star, www.jasminestar.com

Fine Featherheads
www.finefeatherheads.com
Photography: Kate Broussard, Soulshots Photography
www.soulshotsphoto.com

Flavia Carolina, Versa Artistry
www.versaartistry.com
Photography: Heather Nan Photography
www.heathernanphoto.com
Yan Photo, www.yanphoto.com

Honor Kristie, Home Heart Craft
www.homeheartcraft.com

Jemma Grace
www.jemmagrace.com

Jordan Byers
www.jordanbyers.blogspot.com
Photography: Tec Petaja, www.tecpetajaphoto.com

Kayley Heeringa
www.sidewalkready.com
Photography: Kai Heeringa Photography
www.kaiheeringaphotography.com

Ky Wilson, Electric Hairdressing London
www.kycut.co.uk
www.electric-hair.com
Photography: Matt Jones Photography
mattjonesphoto.co.uk

Lana Red Studio
www.lanaredstudio.com

Lesly Lotha, Lazymanxcat
www.lazymanxcat.com
Photography: Urvashi Das
urvashimilliedas@gmail.com

Marie-Pierre Sander
www.studiomariepierre.com

Mindy McKnight
www.cutegirlshairstyles.com

Plum Pretty Sugar
www.plumprettysugar.com
Hairstyling: Makeup 1011, www.1011makeup.com
Katie M, www.katiem.pixpasites.com
Photography: Marisa Holmes
www.marisaholmesblog.com

Suzy Wimbourne Photography
www.suzywimbourne.com

INDEX

ACKNOWLEDGMENTS

The following people have been instrumental in the making of this book, and without them there would be no way I could have possibly put *Braids, Buns, and Twists!* together.

First and foremost I should thank my husband Jim, who has been my pillar of strength in the times when I didn't think I'd get this book finished. I also want to include my mum Jeanette and sister Mary for their constant help, advice, and support.

I want to thank Isheeta, at RotoVision, for her tireless patience throughout, and Diane, my editor, whose constructive criticism has helped make this book so very good. Also, the book's picture researcher, Heidi; Xiaohan, my photographer; and, of course, all of my hair models:

Abigail Schiavello, Adeline Er, An Ly, Arisa Nokubo, Ashleigh Forster, Barbara Rainbird, Carolyn Mach, Delphine Peyriere, Deauvanné, Dorothy Jean Joly, Elly Hanson, Emily Yeo, Hitomi Nakajima, Jane Proust, Jessica Schild, Jessica Tran, Laura Muheim, Michaela Williams, Monica Bowerman, Monica Richmond, Nicole Jeyaraj, Nina Lutz, Olivia English, Ornella Joaquim , Patricia Almario, Riko Ishihata, Ruri Okubo, Sam Colden, Sinead Brady, Sophia Phan, Tanu Vasu, Tash Williams, Teru Morihira, Willa Zheng and Yu Chieh Chen.